The Look
of a
Woman

ERIC PLEMONS

The Look

Facial Feminization Surgery and

# of a

the Aims of Trans- Medicine

Woman

Duke University Press   Durham and London   2017

Interior designed by Courtney Leigh Baker
Cover designed by Amy Ruth Buchanan
Typeset in Whitman and Gill Sans by Copperline

Library of Congress Cataloging-in-Publication Data
Names: Plemons, Eric, [date] author.
Title: The look of a woman : facial feminization
surgery and the aims of trans- medicine / Eric Plemons.
Description: Durham : Duke University Press, 2017. |
Includes bibliographical references and index.
Identifiers:
LCCN 2017001910 (print)
LCCN 2017006457 (ebook)
ISBN 9780822368861 (hardcover : alk. paper)
ISBN 9780822369141 (pbk. : alk. paper)
ISBN 9780822372707 (ebook)
Subjects: LCSH: Male-to-female transsexuals—United
States. | Sex change—United States. | Face—Surgery—
United States. | Surgery, Plastic—United States.
Classification: LCC HQ77.95.U6 P54 2017 (print) |
LCC HQ77.95.U6 (ebook) | DDC 306.76/8—dc23
LC record available at https://lccn.loc.gov/2017001910

Cover art: Annes Bil, *Face Line Drawing*, 2014.
Continuous line drawing; pencil on paper.

For Anne

CONTENTS

Acknowledgments ix

Introduction 1

1 · On Origins
21

INTERLUDE
The Procedures
39

2 · Femininity in
the Clinic
43

INTERLUDE
Celebrate!
67

3 · Cutting as
Caring
71

4 · Recognition
and Refusal
89

INTERLUDE
My Adam's Apple
109

5 · The Operating
Room
113

6 · And After
135

Conclusion 151

Notes 157   References 169   Index 185

ACKNOWLEDGMENTS

There are so many people to thank. First and foremost I am grateful to the surgeons who welcomed me into their busy practices, patiently answering questions and making space for a curious anthropologist in their already hectic days. I am grateful to the surgical patients whose graciousness was truly humbling. Their willingness to tell me their stories and allow me to witness their bodily transformations was profoundly generous, and I hope to have done those stories and transformations a measure of justice here.

I have had the great fortune of working with incredible mentors and collaborators. As a graduate student at the University of California, Berkeley, I am most grateful for the encouragement, enthusiasm, and friendship of my adviser, Cori Hayden, the intellectual wonder and generosity of Lawrence Cohen, the imaginative and expansive thinking of Juana María Rodríguez, and the warmth and inquisitiveness of Charis Thompson. Sharon Kaufman's writing advice and insight were invaluable. I was fortunate to share my time as a graduate student with some wonderful friends who are now my valued colleagues, especially Xochitl Marsilli-Vargas, Katie Hendy, Anthony Stavrianakis, Emily Chua, Nick Bartlett, Kelly Knight, Jeff Schonberg, Liz Kelley, Martine Lappé, and Chris Roebuck, all of whom read and commented on some part of this work over the years. Theresa MacPhail helped talk me over, under, around, and through the process of finishing this book. Laurence Tessier provided the introductions that made this project possible. My work at UC Berkeley was supported by a Dissertation Grant from the Wenner-Gren Foundation and a Dissertation Year Fellowship from Berkeley's Center for the Study of Sexual Cultures.

As a postdoctoral fellow of the University of Michigan Society of Fellows I benefited from the collegiality and support of Tom Fricke, Gayle Rubin, Holly Peters-Golden, Alaina Lemon, Krisztina Fehervary, Helmut Puff, Michael Lempert, Jason De León, Nadine Hubbs, Yasmin Moll, Sarah Besky, Alex Nading, S. E. Kile, Catherine Trundle, and Sebastian Mohr. Liz Roberts was an extraordinary mentor and friend who made Ann Arbor fun and interesting in a million ways. Matthew Chadwick was a terrific research assistant. I am indebted to Donald Lopez Jr. for all he did and continues to do to sustain the Society of Fellows as a network of committed and generous scholars, and to Linda Turner, whose daily work sailed the ship. While at Michigan I came to know the incredibly talented Megan Foldenauer, whose skillful illustrations I am honored to include in this book.

At the University of Arizona I have been welcomed by an excellent group of colleagues and friends, including Diane Austin, Susan Stryker, Susan Shaw, Brian Silverstein, Mark Nichter, Mimi Nichter, Ivy Pike, Eva Hayward, Max Strassfeld, Adela Licona, Francisco Galarte, Russ Toomey, Janelle Lamoreaux, and Monica Casper. I look forward to our continued collaboration.

I am deeply grateful to Ken Wissoker, who saw promise in this project and guided it along, and to Olivia Polk, who helped bring the book to fruition. Many thanks to you, Reader #2, for your multiple rounds of commentary that improved this book in innumerable ways. Thanks, too, to Vincanne Adams for thoughtful and constructive comments in the final rounds.

A version of chapter 1 was published as "Description of Sex Difference as Prescription for Sex Change: On the Origins of Facial Feminization Surgery," *Social Studies of Science* 44(5): 657–79.

LONG BEFORE I KNEW what I wanted to be or make in the world, I had the love and unflagging support of my family. Valerie and Tom Mayer, Doug and Carrie Plemons, Jennifer Plemons, Sam Plemons, Noah Reed, Colin and Kara Snyder, Gloria and Mike Pasche, and Brennan Dougherty, there aren't enough words in the world to express what it means that you all are my home team. Thank you, Carrie McCoy, for being the fiercely loving human to whom I made a promise more than fifteen years ago that I would one day write a book and give your friendship and kindness the acknowledgment it deserves. Thank you, Arturo Baiocchi, for being whip smart, thoughtful, an unmatched conversationalist, and otherwise outstanding company—whether you're across the table or states away. Thank you, Meg Pitman, for the deep love of your friendship. Your humor, tenacity, courage, and care have been more vital to me than you can know. And, though it goes without saying, you are incredibly charming and good-looking. Thank you to my witty, observant, kind, and irrepressible daughter, Jonah. You have been the greatest of life's gifts and are truly my pride and joy. It is a privilege to help you grow into the world, to learn from and with you, and an honor to be your dad.

Finally, I owe my gratitude and more to my wife, Anne. This project has been with us for a long time. You've watched me wrestle with it, love it, curse it, and finally finish it. And there you've always been, ready for anything, moving across the country in support of my goals, filling our home with laughter, friendship, music, and incredible food. You work harder and love harder than anyone I know, throwing your door and heart wide open. You inspire me and challenge me and make me better. You are the most steadfast partner and most deft accomplice a person could have. In you mine is fortune beyond measure.

In weighing the indication for the [genital sex reassignment] operation,
another factor should be considered, namely the physical and especially facial
characteristics of the patient. A feminine habitus, as it existed for instance
in Christine Jorgensen, increases the chances of a successful outcome. A masculine
appearance mitigates against it. Such patient may meet with serious
difficulties later on when he expects to be accepted by society as a
female and lead the life of a woman. —HARRY BENJAMIN, "Transsexualism
and Transvestism as Psycho-Somatic and Somato-Psychic Syndromes," 1954

The argument of this book is a simple one: as ideas shift about the kind of thing that *sex* is, so do the interventions required to change it and the logic of medical practices intended to do so.

Early surgical procedures that aimed to change a person's sex focused on the genitals as the site of a body's maleness or femaleness and took the reconstruction of those organs as the means by which "sex" could be changed, that change always from one binarily conceived sex category to the other. Prospective patients' declared need for genital reconstructive surgery and clinicians' defense of its therapeutic legitimacy anchored the 1950s formulation of *transsexualism* as a psychological condition best treated with physical interventions. While genital surgery remains important to many trans- people, over the past several decades it has been demoted from constituting "sex reassignment surgery" to but one of its possible iterations.[1] No longer exclusively defined by genital form, as treatments for transsexualism once conceived it, now sex is both spread across the entire body—with interventions in chests and breasts, bones, hair, voice, and comportment all made available for purchase—and ever more crucially located outside of the body, in spaces of ongoing social interaction and recognition.

Developed in the mid-1980s, facial feminization surgery (FFS) is a set of bone and soft tissue reconstructive procedures intended to feminize the faces of trans- women. First considered by patients and operating surgeons as an auxiliary procedure in support of the "real" change of sex enacted by genital surgery, now patients who undergo FFS and the surgeons who perform it assert that facial feminization is not a cosmetic operation that simply improves trans- women's appearance; instead FFS itself transforms patients' bodily sex. To claim that facial reconstruction enacts a change of sex is to posit a model of sex—a conceptualization of what and how *sex* is—that departs significantly from the mid-twentieth-century model upon which the diagnosis of *transsexualism* was developed and its genital-centric surgical treatments established. Divorced from an essentialist logic that fixes the truth of sex in discrete anatomical forms, the transformative efficacy of FFS doesn't take place in the closed space of the operating room, nor is it located in the discrete and individual body of the patient herself. Instead FFS works when others recognize and respond to a postoperative patient's face as the face of a woman.

For the patients and surgeons with whom I worked during 2010–11, it was simply obvious that *woman* was not a category constituted by a particular genital anatomy. To be a woman, they asserted, was to be recognized and treated as a woman in the course of everyday life. According to the FFS patients I talked with, if the goal of trans- surgical intervention was to help them realize their identity as women, the most effective site of that intervention was not focused on the generally concealed shape of their genitals but on the visible characteristics of their face. It was *looking* trans- that got FFS patients into trouble on the street. It has been the specter of the masculine-*looking* trans- woman that has fueled proliferating "bathroom bills" across the United States in recent years. For FFS patients, facial surgery was radically transformative because it was a practical acknowledgment that sex was a fundamentally social identity. This is the common sense of FFS: if medical transition is desired to transform a social identity, it must target the social body.

Claims to the transitional efficacy of FFS have been denied and disputed by those who remain committed to a genital definition of sex and thus a genital surgery definition of sex change. Critics argue that "real" sex is genitally defined, or even chromosomally defined, and that no surgery—certainly not facial surgery—can truly change it. Such disputes demonstrate that, in practice, the aims of trans- medicine are not clear, nor are they commonly held among the many players involved in seeking, shaping, and delivering transition-related medical care to trans- Americans. Tensions in the proliferating understandings of the aims of trans- medicine are evident in recent changes to federal, state, and private insurance coverage for "transgender health." Federal regulations passed in 2016 stated that transgender Americans could not be discriminatorily denied coverage for "gender transition services," but stopped short of defining what those services might include.[2] In the absence of an affirmative policy, some insurers understand *transition* broadly, drafting policies that include endocrine interventions, hair removal, voice surgery, chest or breast reconstruction, genital reconstruction, and facial feminization surgeries. Others remain committed to a genital-centric understanding of what transition is and how it might be surgically achieved. The patchwork of covered procedures is not only about money—though funding is always central to debates about American health care. More centrally, varied policies and coverages reflect a prismatic understanding of what it means to transition medically and, more fundamentally, how and under what therapeutic logics trans- medicine is good medicine.

The growing popularity of FFS is emblematic of a shifting landscape in American trans- medicine, one that has been steadily moving away from a narrow focus on genitalia as the site and form of bodily sex and focusing instead on practical enactments of sexual difference that only rarely rely on a congruence between social presentation and genital morphology. The common sense of FFS does not locate surgical efficacy in the atomized, individual body that underwent surgery; instead FFS is understood to work in and through the responses, attributions, and forms of recognition that that body accrues in the interactions of everyday social life. FFS changes the project of surgical sex reassignment by reconfiguring the kind of sex that surgery aims to change.

This book explores how a recognition-based model of sex and of sex change that would have been bafflingly nonsensical when American trans-medicine was institutionalized in the 1960s acquired the force of common sense forty years later. Foregrounding the narratives of patients who undergo FFS and the surgeons who perform their operations, I contend with the history and dynamic present of American trans- medicine to consider what the persistence of some surgical practices and the emergence of others can tell us about how therapeutic logics of trans- medicine are shifting and what *sex* can and could be as a thing made changeable in the surgical clinic. Let me show you what I mean.

Krista had just completed a three-day postoperative exam in Dr. Douglas Ousterhout's office when she eased herself tenderly into a chair opposite me.[3] Fresh white gauze bandages wrapped around the crown of Krista's head, down over her cheeks, and under her chin. The short, stray ends of black sutures were visible at her nasal septum, just under her nostrils, and peeked out from under the dressing on her head in neat rows, tracing her hairline as it descended to her ears. Her eyes and eyelids were blackened and swollen, but the yellow and greenish tones of healing had already begun to appear.

Though Krista was pleased with her recovery progress, she had really hoped to avoid having this surgery. A few years earlier, after seeing Ousterhout give a presentation on "the ten traits of a male face" at a large conference for trans- people, Krista had set about systematically trying to camouflage those traits of her face without the surgery he recommended. She covered her forehead with long, straight-cut bangs. She covered her nose and brow with bulky, nonprescription eyeglasses. She experimented with makeup techniques to minimize the squareness of her jaw. Though she was somewhat satisfied by the results of her efforts, she was simply tired of all the work. "I just couldn't stand the thought of doing all of this for the next twenty years. Just to leave the house? I was thinking about it all the time. My hair had to be perfect. My glasses had to be perfect. It was too much."

Despite her best efforts to cultivate the clothing, makeup, hairstyle, and comportment of the women around whom she lived and worked, other people often saw and responded to Krista as male. But not only male. She was often seen—and treated—as a male who was trying and failing to look female. Krista was sure that her masculine face was spoiling her other efforts at femininity. She felt that she could never truly and simply be accepted as a woman so long as her face constantly threatened to undo her. In one operation lasting just under eleven hours, Ousterhout had rebuilt the bony structure of Krista's forehead, reduced the bridge and tip of her nose, advanced her scalp, reshaped her hairline, reduced the width and squareness of her jaw, shortened the height of her chin, raised her upper lip, removed her thyroid cartilage (Adam's apple), and plumped her lips.

While drowsily recovering from the long hours of anesthetization, Krista had ignored the instruction of the hospital recovery room nurses and tried to stand and walk to the restroom on her own. She rose to her feet and lost consciousness, falling flat on her newly rebuilt face and knocking out a front tooth. Despite being at the very beginning of what would be a long recovery from radical reconstructive surgery as well as an unanticipated root canal, Krista was optimistic. "I'm still puffy," she said, "so I don't really know how I'll end up looking. But all things considered, I think it has gone really well." She had taken the city bus to her appointment that morning. "For the first time in a long time," she explained, "I didn't have to worry about having my bangs just right or wearing just the right pair of glasses. Nobody was looking at me like I was trans-. I looked around and thought, Wow, this is cool." People on that bus were undoubtedly looking at Krista's face covered in gauze bandages, protruding sutures, and colorful bruises. But she found joy in the certainty that whatever they might have seen when they looked at her, the stuff of her maleness was gone. Now she was just another woman on the way to see her plastic surgeon.

Ousterhout developed the procedures now known as facial feminization surgery in the mid-1980s. For decades afterward his name was nearly synonymous with the practice. By the time he retired in 2014, he had performed nearly 1,700 FFS operations—far and away the most of any surgeon in the world. Though he performed other cranio-maxillofacial reconstructive and cosmetic surgeries in his solo private practice, by the mid-1990s FFS patients constituted roughly 80 percent of his thriving practice. During the year I spent observing in his office I met patients who had traveled from Canada, New Zealand, England, Wales, the Netherlands, Germany, India, and Japan to see him. Rumors of his impending retirement increased his caseload as hopeful patients booked appointments just under the wire.

When I met Ousterhout for the first time, he explained FFS as a procedure whose necessity for trans- women was both commonsensical and self-evident. His explanation was delivered, in part, with the use of a *Bloom County* comic depicting three cartoon characters pulling out the waistbands of their underwear and looking down at their (cartoon) genitalia. He slid the image across his desk with a wide grin on his face. "You don't walk down the street looking in everyone's pants before you decide what sex they are. You look at their face," he explained plainly. The absurdity of the comic helped to punctuate his claim; it was so obvious that even cartoon characters knew it. If what a trans- woman ultimately wants from the medicosurgical interventions grouped under the sign of "transition" is to become a woman, then, Ousterhout asserted with absolute certainty, the most dramatic and meaningful change she can undergo is not focused on her genitalia or other hidden parts of her body but on that part that others see the most: her face. Though he did not purport to be offering anything so grand as a *theory* of sex or gender, the ability of this story, and ultimately of FFS, to make sense as a sex-changing intervention certainly depended on one.

Ousterhout's just-so story about what and how "woman" was constituted was one that he fervently believed. So did Krista and the thousands of trans-women that Ousterhout and a handful of other American FFS surgeons had operated on over the past thirty years. Administrators of European gender clinics began incorporating FFS into their holistic health care programs for trans- women in the late 1990s, and a growing number of clinicians from around the world now name avoiding FFS as one reason to start young trans- girls on testosterone blockers before pubertal bone structure changes begin.[4] But as self-evident and commonsensical as the story of sex-as-social-recognition can seem inside the surgical clinic, it is not one that would have always made sense.

When American clinicians conceptualized the diagnosis of transsexualism in the 1950s, they operationalized the emergent distinctions between bodily sex and social gender to define the transsexual as a person who experienced a mismatch between the two. Transsexualism, wrote the pioneering physician Harry Benjamin (1954:220) in 1954, "denotes the intense and often obsessive desire to change the entire sexual status including the anatomical structure. While the male transvestite *enacts* the role of woman, the transsexualist wants to *be* one and *function* as one, wishing to assume as many of her characteristics as possible, physical, mental and sexual." According to this foundational clinical model, the primary thing that a transsexual person (at that time *transsexual* referred almost exclusively to trans- women) wanted and needed in order to be "physically, mentally, and sexually" a woman was reconstructive genital surgery. Though many trans-women continue to value and prioritize genital surgery, a lot has changed about trans- medicine since the 1950s.

ENACTING TRANS- THERAPEUTICS

I use the term *trans- therapeutics* to describe the sets of implicit assumptions and explicit claims that underwrite trans- medicine as a beneficial and therapeutic practice. Trans- therapeutics are the logical frameworks within which various interventions come to make sense as "good trans- medicine." Like all treatment logics, trans- therapeutics link understandings of origins (What is the nature of the concern for which trans- people seek surgical interventions, or the aim toward which particular interventions are attuned?), treatment rationales (Which interventions are appropriate responses to that concern or aim?), and outcome measures (How will we know if those interventions adequately addressed that concern or met their intended aim?). These questions and their answers work together to determine the kind of thing *trans-* is as a clinical object that can organize particular clinical interventions; they shape it as a kind of body project to which particular interventions seem to naturally and rationally correspond. The assertion that facial reconstruction constitutes an enactment of surgical womanhood relies on a particular configuration of trans- therapeutics—a claim about how, why, and by what means facial surgery is good trans- medicine.

Trans- therapeutics change because ideas about sex and gender change. So do ideas about *trans-* as a term that animates medical practice. So do technical capacities and institutional wills to respond to claims for medicosurgical services in the name of trans- medicine. Changes in trans- therapeutics matter because they determine the kinds of care that trans- people can receive, how that care is organized, and thus what kinds of medically mediated bodies are possible and what kinds are not. How did the claim articulated by Krista and her surgeon that a trans- woman can change sex by surgically reconstructing her face—a claim that would have made no sense in the 1950s terms in which transsexualism was formulated—acquire a rhetoric of self-evidence in the mid-1990s? What kind of sex is this? What can the growing popularity of FFS and other nongenital interventions help us to understand about American trans- medicine and the shifting understandings of sex and gender on which it depends? One of the primary aims of this book is to attend to the conditions under which FFS has been increasingly incorporated into contemporary trans- therapeutics and what its growing popularity can tell us about how that therapeutic logic is changing.

The medical anthropologist and science studies scholar Annemarie Mol (2002:vii) has argued that rather than treating clinical diagnoses as naturally given entities to which forms of intervention respond, it is through practices of intervention that medicine "enacts the objects of its concern and treatment." The things that medical actors do with their hands and instruments, the studies they design and questions they ask, and the services that patients request bring clinical entities into being in particular ways

(Mol 2002; Mol and Berg 1994). It is through practices that contested ideas about sex, gender, and trans- bodies are materialized into action and incited into speech; they move from abstract concepts into material bodies and observable techniques. What are trans- people asking from the surgeons whose services they seek? What is the nature of the sex that FFS aims to alter? Under what model of trans- therapeutics can FFS be said to work? What work does it do?

In my focus on the productivity of patient interventions, I adopt Mol's (2002) analytic of enactment. Emerging from scholarship in science and technology studies focused on the daily practices by which experts make knowledge, a focus on enactment is committed to ethnographic specificity. It foregrounds contextualized doing—the things that are happening in examination rooms and operating rooms—to better understand the specific conditions under which claims to knowledge are produced and come to have the force of fact. Enactment insists on specific actions unfolding in time and space (Mol and Law 1994). It allows me to begin from the premise that neither woman nor femininity nor trans- medicine is a singular or stable thing for which FFS is a discrete kind of response. All of these are enacted, brought into being as things in the world through the use of particular practices employed by patients and their surgeons.

ACCOUNTING FOR SHIFTS IN CONCEPTUALIZATIONS OF SEX AND GENDER

Ideas about how and as what *sex* is defined have changed considerably since the 1950s, when American sexological and psychological researchers created clinical distinctions between physical sex and psychosocial gender. Reflecting American anxieties after World War II about the place of men and women in economic, family, and political life, their research aimed to control and treat forms of sexual and psychosexual difference by rendering that difference classifiable in a raft of new diagnoses, including transsexualism (Downing et al. 2015; Irvine 1990; Karkazis 2008; Rudacille 2005). The definition and divisions of physical sex from psychosocial gender that emerged from that clinical research did not stay confined to the clinic. The conceptual separation of sex (conceived as bodily form and matter) from gender (conceived as a set of power-laden social roles and relations largely and variously derived from the material forms of sex) became a central premise upon which late twentieth-century feminist politics, scholarship, and activism was based.

In the 1990s, however, the philosopher Judith Butler confronted American feminism with an "imminent critique" of the terms by which feminism had been organized. In her iconic book *Gender Trouble* (1990) Butler questioned the role that heterosexuality and "natural" femininity had in constituting the identity category "woman" upon which feminist politics depended. Enmeshed in a Foucauldian concern with the regulatory power of sexuality and a psychoanalytic approach to understanding sexual difference and subject formation, Butler sought not only to denaturalize gender—this was the project of social constructionist feminism of the 1970s and 1980s—but also to denaturalize and historicize sex.

Adapting a linguistic framework developed by John Austin (1962), Butler advanced a performative theory of gender, arguing that gender (masculinity or femininity) does not flow from a naturally sexed bodily essence but is instead made to seem essential through continued acts of repetition (what Butler, after Derrida [1988], called "citation"). Thus masculinity and femininity are not inherent properties of bodies or of persons. Instead individuals become recognizable to themselves and others as instances of masculinity or femininity by doing things that are already understood in those terms, by citing gendered norms. Sex and sexual difference are, Butler argued, produced the same way. Male and female bodies come to seem opposed or mutually exclusive because of the way we talk about them, study them, place emphasis on distinctions rather than commonalities, and use metaphors that leverage existing understandings and values of masculinity and femininity to understand biological or genetic—or in the case of FFS osteological—processes.[5] As such, she argued, ideas about how sex difference is constituted are themselves among the most entrenched products of citational gender practices, making sex as unstable and contingent a category as gender. They are mutually reinforcing and co-constitutive: sex/gender.

One of the reasons Austin's framework was so generative for Butler is that, rather than engaging solely with language, Austin was concerned with communication. While language can be studied as a closed system with logics and structures unto itself, communication requires production and reception, and, crucially, it happens in a context. Central to Austin's formulation of performativity (and so key to Derrida's critique and Butler's adaptation) is a concern with the existing rules and norms of social life that determine what can be communicated, by whom, to whom, and under what circumstances. Like communicative language, in Butler's view, sex/gender is determined in and through relations of authority; it is enabled and constrained by power. In acts of citation, reception, and recognition, forms of power are negotiated, making some claims to sexed/gendered being possible and others impossible.

In a performative model citation and reception of sex/gender norms are predicated on recognition, the act of exchange by which we come into being for ourselves and each other. Social norms and expectations determine *who* is recognizable *to whom* and *as what*. What kinds of bodies are recognizable as female bodies? What kinds as male? If we accept that sex, as Butler and others have argued, has a history, then it is clear that there is no single answer to these questions. Instead what kinds of bodies and thus what kinds of persons might be recognized as female change across time and place, in relation to who is looking and what they are looking for. The intersubjectivity of this model is crucial. If recognition is the means through which sex/gender becomes materialized and naturalized, then the conditions of recognition are the conditions of gender: I am a man when I am recognized as a man. It is precisely this kind of productive recognition that animated the practice of facial feminization surgery. Surgeons and patients were attuned to the promise that facial surgery could make transwomen recognizable to others as the women they knew themselves to be. The efficacy of FFS as a sex-changing surgery was claimed in and through acts of recognition.

I do not lay out this framework in order to stage a performative reading of FFS. Indeed, following Butler one would argue that all gendered acts—especially ones so self-consciously oriented toward the production of normative gender—are performative. To argue that FFS is among them would not provide much insight or attend to the specificity of FFS practice. Instead I read FFS as the material result of integrating a performative model of sex/gender into a plan for trans- medicine. When sex is understood as a product of recognition, then surgery explicitly aimed at altering the terms of that recognition becomes self-evidently and commonsensically a sex-changing intervention. Though surgeons and patients did not describe their shared theory of sex/gender as performative, they articulated its main claims as the common sense that underwrote the transformative power of FFS. The trans- therapeutics of FFS were performative.

Because assertions of sex-as-recognition were central to the patients and surgeons with whom I worked and because the claim to FFS efficacy depended on them, rather than relying on an *analytics* of performativity, I treat the model itself as an ethnographic object—a move that Stefan Helmreich (2011:136) has called working "*athwart theory*: thinking of theory neither as set above the empirical nor as simply deriving from it, but as crossing the empirical transversely." For Helmreich, theory is "at once an abstraction as well as a thing in the world; theories constantly cut across and complicate our paths as we navigate forward in the 'real' world" (136). I treat the theory of performative gender—the assertion of sex-as-recognition—as a historically particular style of thought whose wide-reaching influence includes a framing and articulation of trans- therapeutics that was not possible before the 1990s.[6] It is by assigning productive power to acts of recognition and valuing the sociality of sex by emphasizing the productivity of social recognition that FFS is understood not as complementary to a trans- woman's transition but the very means by which woman comes to be. The performative intervention interrupts the distinction between "enacting the role of woman" and "being a woman" that Benjamin initially used to distinguish transvestism from transsexualism. In a performative framework sex and gender are intersubjective and irreducibly social things—a distinctly different kind of subject and different kind of sex and gender than the biologically universal, anatomical, and atomistic model of sex that first conceived the transsexual as a person whose desire to be a woman necessitated transformative genital surgery.

To be clear, I am not suggesting that the theorization of performative sex/gender was *causally* responsible for the growth of FFS and other forms of nongenital trans- body modification, nor that scores of trans- women are marching into medical offices waving *Gender Trouble* over their head or speaking of their transition in the terms of high theory. I am arguing that arriving as it did into the ripe critical space opened by social constructionism and an emerging skepticism of scientific and medical authority, the central elements of gender performativity became discursive resources by which claims to the nature of sex and gender—and thus the nature and form of trans- therapeutics—could emerge as such in the 1990s in ways that they could not and had not before.[7] Theories describe the world and also become things in the world that produce affects and effects.

The French feminist theorist Anne Emmanuelle Berger (2014:78) has argued that "gender theory is not a pure conceptual construction, that it is also a cultural artifact, and that it has to be treated as such, that we have to raise the question of its contexts of production and reception, its modes of existence, and its rhythms of circulation" (see also Valentine 2007). I take up Berger's provocation to consider how the premises of gender performativity have shaped claims about the nature of sex and gender and the medical practices intended to intervene in them. The claim that sex is made real in and through acts of intersubjective recognition—that sex is performative—is the animating logic of FFS; it underwrites a trans- therapeutics within which FFS as a sex-changing technology acquires the force of common sense.

Of course the explanation of trans- medicine as focused on nongenital body parts and as being oriented toward a goal of recognition was not solely produced by a shift in discursive resources. Its emergence in the 1990s has a great deal to do with changes in how trans- medicine was administered and the kinds of narratives trans- people could tell about their lives that had been foreclosed in the previous decades by gatekeeping diagnostic protocols that trained a focus on genitals and genital surgery.

FROM "WRONG BODY" TO "INVISIBLE ME"

The practice of FFS begins at the first surgical consultation and ends at the last postoperative checkup. But the conditions of its possibility—the political, institutional, and conceptual histories that led to the emergence and continued popularization of FFS—stretch to the earliest moments of American trans- medicine and portend shifts to come. The historian Joanne Meyerowitz (2002) has argued that the shift of trans- medicine from university-based clinics to private practice in the late 1970s and 1980s is the event that has had the greatest impact on trans- health care in the United States. In making the move from research hospitals to private practice, trans- medicine was part of a massive wave of privatization of American medicine in the 1980s. In for-profit trans- medicine, as in other medical specialties, patients qua consumers were newly empowered—and expected—to direct their own health care decisions (Balint and Shelton 1996). While this meant a welcome break from the paternalism and restriction that had characterized university clinic programs in the 1960s and 1970s, it also introduced new problems of access. Many trans- people were unable to afford expensive specialty surgeries. Others paid a small number of surgeons who provided a much-needed service in exchange for a very handsome fee, opening questions about whether surgeons' work was driven by a will to generously help people in need or to exploit and profit from that need (Morreim 1995).

The ethical contentiousness of care versus profit was especially debated in regard to the exponential growth of elective surgery in the 1980s and 1990s (Blum 2003, 2005; Bordo 1997; Gilman 1998; Morgan 1991).[8] A growing consumer commodity, elective surgery was marketed to achieve the American values of individual improvement, self-actualization, and self-esteem that were crucial for a strong economy and fundamental to the robust nationalism of the cold war era (Edmonds 2009; Gilman 1998; Haiken 1997; Meyerowitz 2002; Serlin 2004). Political, economic, and popular shifts toward the neoliberal values of personal responsibility and market-based solutions to social problems in the 1980s and a rapidly specializing medical profession (Starr 1982) helped to create an American health care system that celebrated individual choice and freedom (Mol 2008; Patton 2010), making each of us responsible for cultivating the self-actualization that comes from living as fully realized individuals in "healthy" bodies (Briggs and Hallin 2007; Rabinow 1996; Rose 2007).

Once the hallmark of transsexual self-narrative, "wrong body discourse"— the explanation of trans- embodiment as, for example, being a woman trapped in a man's body—was adopted by people seeking surgical self-realization of many kinds (Frangos 2006). Thin people trapped in fat bodies (Bordo 1993; Throsby 2008), attractive people trapped in ugly bodies (Davis 2003a; Huss-Ashmore 2000), and young people trapped in old bodies (Frost 2005; Holliday and Taylor 2006) turned to a market saturated by surgeons whose procedures promised to make mismatched selves and bodies into harmonious pairs (Gilman 1999; Shilling 1993). Immersed in a context of surgical self-optimization and newly empowered to direct the processes and components of their own transitions, many trans- Americans in the 1990s embraced a new narrative about what surgery was meant to do. Rather than moving them from one "wrong body" to a binarily opposed "right body," surgery could be for trans- people what it was for others: a means of individual self-actualization, a way to make an "invisible me" visible to others. Disaggregated from narratives of pathology and increasingly available in a fee-for-service, consent-based, and patient-centered treatment model, the popularization of FFS in the mid-1990s depended upon these dynamics; it was part of an American trans- medicine tuned to a newly defined outcome of self-fulfillment and personal authenticity.

Of course medically mediated self-fulfillment is not available to everyone. Medical transition can be very expensive, and the high cost of surgical procedures puts them out of reach of many who desire them. Even more expensive than genital reconstruction, and with only very recent and exceedingly rare insurance coverage, FFS is a luxury available only to the resourced few. I take up these critiques at length in chapter 4.

What distinguishes FFS from other trans- surgeries is the primary role it gives to the social life of the body. While an individual body undergoes surgical interventions, the change that FFS enacts takes place irreducibly between people. Perhaps nowhere is this made clearer than in the imaginary scene in which Ousterhout explains the goal of FFS: "If, on a Saturday morning, someone knocks at the door and you wake up and get out of bed with messy hair, no makeup, no jewelry, and answer the door, the first words you'll hear from the person standing there are 'Excuse me, Ma'am.'"

Other FFS surgeons I interviewed narrated similar scenes, and many patients reproduced them when describing their hopes for postsurgical life. Rachel fantasized about walking into a store and having the clerk ask, "Can I help you, Miss?" Gretchen imagined sitting on an airplane without having to endure the reproachful stares and palpable discomfort of the passenger seated next to her. Tracy hoped that she would no longer "scare small children" when she walked down the street. It was in moments at the doorstep, in the shop, on the airplane, or on the street that FFS patients would know that the procedure had worked, that it had done what they'd hoped it would. It was in the "miss," the "madam," and the not-looking-twice that their womanhood would be enacted.

Some people—including some of the FFS patients I talked with—might consider such scenes to be instances of passing. *Passing* is a term with a fraught history in U.S. racial and sexual politics (Cooley and Harrison 2012; Ginsberg 1996; Hobbs 2014; Robinson 1994). For some trans- people the term is contentious because it implies deception. Some trans- women object to the language of passing because, they argue, to say that someone passes as a woman is to affirm that woman is not a category to which she rightfully belongs. The author and activist Julia Serano (2007:176–82) has argued that passing is often used to describe the actions and efforts of a person whose body and behavior are being scrutinized, thereby obscuring the active role of those scrutinizing her. This singular focus, Serano writes, creates a double standard in which the gender work of non-trans- people—whom she calls *cisgender* or *cissexual*—is solidified as natural and effortless while trans- people's gender is maintained as artificial and deliberate.[9]

Rather than a project of passing, FFS is more productively read as a project oriented by an aim of recognition. Though no less complicated, approaching trans- body projects, especially FFS, as aiming for recognition offers a set of analytic tools and stakes that move beyond questions of authenticity and artifice, truth and falseness, duplicity and strategy that often structure discussions of passing. Theories of recognition from Hegel to Honneth share a fundamental understanding of the individual not as a bounded and atomistic subject but as one formed in and through relations with others. They focus on the dynamic productivity of intersubjective interaction. Recognition is fundamental to a performative model of sex/gender and, as the scenes above attest, is central to the imagined and actual means through which FFS does its work.

A shift from passing to recognition allows us to attend to what happens when a trans- woman's efforts toward being recognized as a woman are refused. Refusals of her womanhood do not only negate her efforts toward desirable recognition; they also produce forms of recognition that she does not desire. In this way recognition is productive, but not always affirmative.[10] Being recognized in an unwelcome way can be destructive and dangerous (McQueen 2015). This kind of unwelcome and "undoing" recognition (Butler 2004) can happen interpersonally—when, instead of "miss," the shop owner mutters something hateful and threatening, in relation to the state when facial surgery is irrelevant to questions of legal sex, and politically when other trans- people read some kinds of recognition as liberatory and others as dangerously conciliatory. The dynamic and entangled relations of recognition allow us to see FFS as suspended in tensions with each of these in ways that "pass/not pass" does not. When FFS works (or not), it does more than change one person's face.

WRITING ME IN

It would be difficult to overestimate the role that my being a trans- man has played in this research. It has shaped how the project was conceived as well as the kinds of data I was able to collect.[11] This acknowledgment is not meant to flatten or trivialize significant differences between and among people who identify themselves as trans- (transgender, transsexual, trans*, or any one of many shifting and proliferating terms). The patients I interviewed, talked with, and shared time with had been recognized for most of their lives as boys and men and had come to the surgical clinic looking for surgeons' help to transform their body so they could be recognized—by themselves and others—as the woman they knew themselves to be. Some identified as trans-, some as transgender, some as transsexual. Many talked about these words as relevant to their life or terms with which they related, but they did not explicitly assign them to themselves, and I did not ask them to do so.

I am in a body that has allowed me to think of gender as flexible and malleable. My transition was emotionally exhausting and often excruciating. I hope to never experience such profound self-doubt and self-scrutiny ever again. But the physical ambiguity of that period—the time when my sex could be and was read differently several times in a day or even in the course of a single interaction—was mercifully brief. With some help from twice-monthly testosterone injections, my body facilitated the shift from woman to man that I resolved to make. No surgery was required to enact this shift—though some was certainly desired and eventually undergone. I am a man in every sense of the word that matters to me. And crucially, I am not alone in my claim to manhood. My status as a man—and thus as presumptively male-bodied—is reflected back to me from all directions. Strangers and intimates recognize me as a man. So does the state; the big block M on my driver's license, passport, and birth certificate completes the story of my identity. The coherence of my sexed appearance and identification documents allows me to obtain legal employment, move unimpeded across national borders, and gain access to the myriad privileges of unquestioned white manhood. Considering my story in the abstract, some may contend that I am not in fact a man and that my "real" sex is safely confirmed by my XX chromosomes. Those folks and I are working with different definitions of sex, different ideas about what the word *man* denotes, and that's okay with me. Because my status as a man is recognized and consistently accepted by individuals and institutions, because it blends me in and keeps me safe, I can afford not to care about the opinions of naysayers. I shrug in the shape of that privilege. That there was a significant gap between my story of medical transition and theirs was a fact not lost on the trans- women with whom I spoke during my fieldwork.

Some bodies avail themselves of theories of gendered fluidity and flux, play and performance. Others do not. Some bodies bear signs of distinction that are so strong and so immediately recognizable in the social milieu in which they exist that no dress, no makeup, no mannerisms, no hormones, no deeply felt personal claims can effectively resignify them. In some cases the persons who inhabit such bodies take up their outsider status proudly and to great effect. They relish being physical catalysts for social change and for upsetting a normative gender system that divides and denigrates us all. Other people do not want to be the vanguard for changing the gender system in which they live. They want, like the overwhelming majority of people, to be simply and unquestionably recognized as the man or woman they know themselves to be. But for some bodies this desire is nearly impossible to achieve. The shapes of acceptable femininity are constrained far more than those of acceptable masculinity (Serano 2007). For the trans-women I met in the course of my research, the fact of their face marked the difference between the life they had and the life they wanted.

There are many who object to the surgical impulse, arguing that an often lurid focus on surgery has, for too long, overdetermined trans- as a medical category—both for those trans- people who desire surgical transformation and for those who think and write about trans- lives. While I am sympathetic to that critique and grateful for the creative and vital scholarship that has emerged in its wake, I think it is important to remember that the practice of trans- surgery has gone on uninterrupted in the United States for over six decades. In that time there has not been a single day in which the surgeons who specialize in trans- specific procedures have not been busy at their craft, and not a day when the queue of hopeful patients has disappeared. I am an ethnographer of trans- surgical practice not because surgery defines us as trans- people but because it is so very important to so many of our lives.

Inside the clinic patients' personal stories, rationales for seeking surgery, and theories of trans- embodiment are transformed into a set of plans. Surgeons don't operate on desire or justice or fantasy or redemption or self-actualization or shame or any of the other things that surgeries might mean to trans- people. Surgeons perform procedures on body parts. Those procedures are oriented toward particular goals, nameable transformations that are planned in advance, for a particular reason, and (hopefully) evaluated for their success or failure after the fact. How patients relate to those goals, how they contribute to their formation and make sense of them afterward are intimately linked to the technical work of surgery but are not the same as that work.

Facial feminization surgery is not simply one more way to enact the end goal of woman that was first articulated in and through transsexualism and its genital surgery treatment. It is not the same project focused on a different body part. Instead FFS is animated by a different understanding of what and how sex is. It articulates an alternative therapeutic logic and, by implication, an alternative framing of what trans- medicine aims to do and how and why it aims to do it. In the FFS clinic patients and surgeons assert a trans- therapeutics centered on a body enlivened and invested with socially particular meanings. They enact a surgical logic that moves sex/gender out of individual bodies and into the social space between people, where the performative claim that sex/gender is made real through recognition can be worked into a surgical plan. This project takes the claims of FFS patients seriously—that the fulfillment of their desire for transition can be enacted through facial reconstruction—and contends with the historical, political, and ethical implications of that claim.

But one step at a time.

CHAPTER BY CHAPTER

In the first chapter I explore the origins of FFS in its historical and geographical moment: San Francisco in the early 1980s. By analyzing how Ousterhout's treatment philosophy has changed over time, I show how shifts in ideas about sex and gender and in the delivery of trans- medicine in the dynamic 1990s impacted the way he understood and performed FFS. Initially committed to the genital-centric definition of transsexualism in relation to which FFS was complementary, over time and in consultation with his patients Ousterhout come to understand FFS as itself enacting a change of sex.

In chapter 2 I examine how conflicting models of trans- therapeutics are worked out in the surgical clinic. By analyzing one initial patient consultation in Ousterhout's office and another in the office of a plastic surgeon, Joel Beck, I argue that these divergent clinical strategies are indicative not only of shifts in trans- treatment paradigms but of broader trends in the ways Americans use surgery. No longer limited by the "wrong body" model of pathology that structured trans- medicine between the 1960s and 1980s, by the first decades of the twenty-first century trans- people could join the ranks of millions of Americans who sought surgery in order to manifest their true self. This change in treatment philosophy multiplies what it means for trans- surgical interventions to work, thereby implicating a shift in the aims and logics of trans- medicine.

In chapter 3 I look at the ethical history of American trans- medicine as a distinct "geography of care" and show how it continues to bear on the clinical present. Surgeons' efforts to frame their work with trans- patients in ethical and affective terms both respond to the fact of poor trans- health care and leverage that legacy to distinguish "good" surgeons from "bad." Described as an act of friendship, generosity, and deific repair that patients reciprocated with gratitude, loyalty, and individualized moralistic praise, facial feminization surgery was an act of restitutive intimacy whose status as such depended upon the elision of the financial transaction between doctor and patient. As surgeons claimed to care for their trans- patients for "all the right reasons," their ability to surgically enact woman depended in part on the cultivation of affect as a vital surgical technique.

In chapter 4 I move out of the surgical clinic to look at contexts of recognition in which the claims to performative womanhood that surgeons and patients name common sense are explicitly refused. Rather than an instance of passing, I suggest recognition is a more productive way to understand the aims of FFS and one that allows a consideration of the effects of FFS in scales other than face-to-face interaction. The personal recognition of belonging and authentic identity that FFS patients seek is contentious for some trans- women who claim that rather than individual recognition as normatively female, what they need is political recognition as an identity group. Advocating collective refusal of the narrow norms that constrain sex/gender subjectivity, these critics argue that FFS costs trans- women more than they should bear. The personal and face-to-face recognition that FFS patients seek is also refused by the state, whose definition of sex and surgical sex-reassignment remains centered on genital anatomy. By engaging the complexities of recognition over the dichotomy of pass/no pass, I argue that we are better able to contend with the effects of FFS beyond the individuals who undergo it.

In chapter 5 I go into the operating room to watch FFS get done. In that space I was confronted with tensions between the abstract tools I had for thinking about sex/gender embodiment and the visceral materiality of reconstructive surgery. Interspersing detailed field notes of one patient's operation within an analytic exploration of the place that trans- bodies have occupied in gender theory, I explore tensions between the body in books and the body on the table. It is ethnography that provides a meeting place between the two, insisting that it is in the situated practices of living that bodies, like ideas, acquire potential and meet their limits. Cutting, sawing, and suturing are examples of potential and limit, both for me and for the patient whose deeply intimate transformation I witnessed.

In chapter 6 I ask what happens to patients after surgery. Exploring the narratives of three patients—one directly following surgery who is imagining its ultimate effects, one whose surgery is considered an unqualified success, and one who finds that FFS did not do for her what she hoped it would—multiplies questions of how and for whom FFS works, unsettling any simple narrative of what this surgery can do. In the end I think through some ways that a shift to intersubjective and recognition-based definitions of sex/gender are influencing medical practice and how we think of transtherapeutics in America today.

I · On Origins

The classification of individuals into dichotomous sex categories inevitably
involves cultural work made possible by a history of definitional acts.
—STEVEN EPSTEIN, *Inclusion*, 2007

BEGINNING BEFORE THE BEGINNING

Douglas Ousterhout had just completed a general surgery residency at the
University of Michigan when, in 1970, he packed up his life in Ann Arbor
and moved to Palo Alto to begin a plastic surgery residency at Stanford
University. "Before I started at Stanford," he explained, "I told them I didn't
want to work with the gender program. I had heard what Don Laub was
doing there, and I wasn't interested in working with transsexual patients."
In the early 1970s virtually every plastic surgeon in the United States was
aware of the new programs being established at universities across the
country that were offering surgical services to a growing group of patients
diagnosed as transsexual.

The first of these clinics opened at Johns Hopkins University in 1966,
the year after Ousterhout graduated from medical school. Largely funded
by private individual and institutional grants from the Erickson Educational
Foundation,[1] the Hopkins clinic served as an early model for the develop-

ment of similar university-based clinics across North America, ushering in a brief period in the mid-1960s to late 1970s that the historian Susan Stryker (2008:93) has called "the 'Big Science' period of transgender history." Despite ongoing controversies among psychologists and medical doctors over what kinds of medical and surgical treatments should be offered to people newly understood to be suffering from transsexualism or gender dysphoria—if indeed any such treatments should be offered at all (Reay 2014)—at least a dozen university-based gender clinics were operating in the United States by 1979 (Restack 1979).[2] Stanford University's Gender Dysphoria Program (GDP) opened in 1968 under the direction of Dr. Donald Laub, a plastic surgeon, and would prove to be one of the most influential programs in the country.

During his time as a plastic surgery resident at Stanford, Ousterhout's request to avoid working with Laub's GDP patients was granted, for the most part. He was never trained in the techniques used in genital sex-reassignment procedures—the operations most commonly associated with transsexual surgical interventions and for which Laub would become quite well known—but Ousterhout did see GDP patients in postoperative rounds and provided postsurgical care appropriate to his status as a resident. "I didn't have any real reason not to like them," he explained of the GDP patients. "I think that like most people at the time, I just didn't know anything about transsexuals, and I didn't really want to know." After leaving Stanford, Ousterhout turned his attention to craniofacial reconstructive surgery and thought his encounters with transsexual patients were behind him. But his connection to Stanford plastic surgery and the rapidly changing landscape of transmedicine in the United States would bring trans- patients to his attention again nearly a decade later.

As quickly as they had been established, American gender clinics began to close down in the late 1970s. Despite its central role in the institutionalization of trans- medicine and the many technical innovations produced by its surgeons, the Stanford Gender Dysphoria Program closed its doors in 1980, when, like many chief surgeons in gender clinics around the country, Laub left academic medicine for private practice. (He continued to operate on trans- people as patients of Gender Dysphoria Program, Inc., now a private clinic located across the street from Stanford's campus.)[3]

In 1982, two years after the Stanford program severed relations with the university, a former patient named Candace returned to see the surgeon who had performed her genital sex-reassignment surgery (GSRS) some years before. Despite the profound change that GSRS had enacted in her body and sense of self, Candace found that its transformative power was limited to her body alone. Though the fact of her restructured genitalia constituted her as a woman medically and legally, socially it made no change in her life at all. Like many women Candace had gone to great lengths to cultivate a desirably feminine body: she wore her hair long and well styled, and she made strategic choices in clothing and makeup. She had begun what would be a lifelong regimen of hormonal therapy, undergone electrolysis to remove her facial and body hair, and devoted considerable time to retraining her voice and comportment. Despite her best efforts, however, others still saw and reacted to her not as the woman she knew she was but as a man who was trying—but failing—to look like a woman. She endured insults and stares and felt the weight of disdain directed at those whose bodily presentations deviate from the norm. The fact of her new female genitalia—the bodily metonym of sex difference whose transformation is often believed to instantiate if not to define "sex change"—was secreted away behind the bounds of propriety in social life: no one knew it was there. But they did see her face. It was clear to Candace that her face was the problem. She had a man's face. No amount of makeup or decoration could hide it. She returned to her plastic surgeon, wondering if anything could be done. Her surgeon turned to Ousterhout.

By that time Ousterhout had established himself as a distinguished cranio-maxillofacial surgeon.[4] After leaving Stanford years before, he completed a prestigious fellowship with the renowned craniofacial surgeon Paul Tessier in Paris and then returned to California, where he helped to found the Center for Craniofacial Anomalies at the University of California, San Francisco, Medical Center. Prior to Candace's request, Ousterhout had never thought about skulls as being male or female, masculine or feminine. "Here I had been operating at UCSF for several years," Ousterhout explained, "and I had never thought about the differences between a boy's and a girl's skull." Ousterhout's work as a cranio-maxillofacial surgeon had been guided by the directive to make pathologically abnormal skulls and faces into "normal" ones. And up to that point "normal" had not been a sexed or gendered category.

Still ambivalent about working with transsexual patients, Ousterhout was intrigued by Candace's problem and drawn to the technical challenge her case presented. Treating her offered him the chance to do something new. Whatever technical skills might be necessary, the first step was a definitional one: at that point, as a surgical category, "the female face" did not yet exist.

This chapter begins with the story of how facial feminization surgery was developed in the early 1980s and ends with an accounting of how Ousterhout's FFS practice looked when I began working in his office in 2010. In the early years Ousterhout considered facial surgery a cosmetic procedure that was auxiliary to the transsexual patient's primary treatment of genital surgery: genital surgery changed her sex; facial surgery made her appear more congruously female. Over time, however, his opinion about the kind of change FFS enacted began to shift. In conversation with his patients, more and more of whom sought FFS either before GSRS or in lieu of it, Ousterhout began to understand FFS not as supplementary to the change of sex effected by genital surgery but as enacting a change of sex in and of itself. It was when others recognized a trans- woman as a woman that she truly became one; the shape of her genitals was simply irrelevant most of the time. By the mid-1990s Ousterhout had come to understand facial reconstruction surgery as enabling a much more meaningful transformation in the lives of trans- women than any other surgical procedure could. Not a private nor a genital affair, FFS was both influenced by and provided a medical model for thinking sex/gender as an effect of social exchange and intersubjective recognition, a shift that would ultimately offer an alternative way to interpret the goal of transition and the place of medicine within it.

HOW TO MAKE A FEMININE FACE, IN THREE STEPS

Some three decades after he'd originally set out to devise a series of procedures to make Candace's male face into a female face, Ousterhout told me that his research had involved three main steps. First, he needed to determine where sex was located in the face—which bone and soft tissue structures marked meaningful differences between male and female—in order to know precisely where to intervene. Finding no help from medical sources for which a wide variety of anatomical forms fall into the unsexed category of "normal," he turned to a tradition of scholarship that had long been interested in what skull variations might demonstrate about human difference: physical anthropology. He found cues to sex distinction in the now highly contested methods by which early twentieth-century physical and forensic anthropologists assigned sex to human remains. Second, he needed to ascertain how to quantify the sex differences anthropologists had identified so that he could surgically reproduce them. He found these quantifications in an early twentieth-century orthodontic study conducted on schoolchildren at the University of Michigan. Third, he needed to determine how to turn this information on sites and forms of difference into a feasible surgical plan. For this practical application he visited a collection of skulls amassed in the early twentieth century and housed at the Dugoni School of Dentistry at the University of the Pacific in San Francisco. After this three-step research was complete, Ousterhout worked across and knitted relations between these three very different types of source material in order to produce two things: a definition of a distinctly female face and a set of surgical procedures he could use to produce it. These procedures would become known as facial feminization surgery.

Defining the term *feminine* that lies at the heart of the project of facial feminization surgery is no easy task. Sometimes a biological category anchored to the genes and hormones of the female, and sometimes an aesthetic category defined by desirable beauty, *feminine* is a term in which biological femaleness and aesthetic desirability collapse. *Female, feminine,* and *femininity* are terms whose definitions are deeply tied to racial notions of the normal and ideal body, the normal and ideal woman. The story of facial feminization surgery is entwined in these powerful methodological, political, and epistemological histories. Like all trans- medicine, the practice of FFS materializes into action and incites into speech contested ideas about sexed bodies; it defines sexual difference as a condition of devising strategies to produce it. When conceptualizations of sex and gender change, so do the medical interventions intended to respond to them.

Step One: Physical Anthropology

When he began to search for the craniofacial morphology of sexual difference, Ousterhout joined a long and contentious legacy of American research that has sought to understand the relationship between skeletal features and forms of social difference. The field of physical anthropology was established in the United States in the first decades of the twentieth century.[5] Reflecting contemporary social and political anxieties, early research on racial difference and the place of women in economic and political life was guided by the idea that social differences between groups were the result of—and could therefore be observed in—physical differences in the bodies of group members. Most often associated with naturalist studies of race in the eighteenth and nineteenth centuries, measurements of the skull and face remained a primary focus of research until the methods of what is now often called "scientific racism" fell out of favor following World War II. Still the influence of this scholarship lives on in many forms, including the claims to sexual difference that it helped to produce and the material collections of skeletal matter on which those claims are based (Blakey 1987; Fabian 2010; Gould 1981; Haraway 1989; Lindqvist 1997; Van Wyhe 2004).

Ousterhout turned to physical anthropology because anatomical and medical atlases—the typical resources of the reconstructive surgeon—do not identify distinctly male and female skeletal forms. So long as they enable people to function healthfully, doctors rarely pay attention to the ways bones vary in size and shape from person to person. Physical and forensic anthropologists, however, pay a great deal of attention to this kind of variation. These practitioners use differences in the size, shape, and quality of particular bones to distinguish a number of characteristics about an individual, including that individual's sex—a category that until quite recently in archaeological scholarship had only two options: male or female.[6] Skulls have been central to studies of skeletal sex distinction.

There is no such thing as a skull that exhibits sex characteristics alone. Though researchers may treat categories of interest such as sex, age, nutrition, race, or population group as distinct variables, in fact these aspects of any given body are inextricably entangled; they form and inform each other. It is not possible to ascertain the sex of a given skull without also considering the age at which the person died, for example, because the age of a skeleton largely determines the extent to which sex-differentiating characteristics are present (Meindl et al. 1985). Similarly, placing a skull into a sex category also requires an understanding of the race or population group to which a skull belongs.[7] In short, sex, like race and age, is a contingent category; its expression is never independent of other biological and environmental factors that influence skeletal characteristics (Gere 1999; Joyce 2005). When producing an ostensibly neutral model of a female or male skull, characteristics that might exhibit such things as race and age are not gone; their irrelevance to the didactic aim of the model only makes them seem to disappear.

To make matters even more complex, human male and female bodies "share about 95% of the total range of [physical] variation," meaning that male and female bodies are far more alike than different and that nearly every bodily characteristic found in an individual placed in one sex category can be found in an individual placed in another (St. Hoyme and İşcan

1989:59). Though anthropological scholarship has continually stressed these complexities and contingencies, unfamiliar readers committed to and invested in the idea that human bodies come in mutually exclusive and sexually dimorphic forms don't always contend with their intricacies. Taking the project of transsexual transition seriously—that the process facilitates the transformation of one sexed body to *the* other—Ousterhout was looking for a distinctively female skull, and in his reading early twentieth-century physical anthropology supplied it.

As Siobhan Somerville (2000) and others have argued, early twentieth-century scholarship on racial and sexual classification considered the white body the norm from which racially marked bodies diverged. This foundational assumption animated the early anthropological sources that Ousterhout consulted and, as I describe in the next section, also populated the data from which his FFS figures emerged. (For a more detailed account of this research, see Plemons 2014.) Though not intentionally so, the model "female skull" that resulted from Ousterhout's research was a distinctly northern European skull, bearing the historical legacy and practical burdens of its creation. A key part of that historical legacy is the refusal that it is historical at all. Instead a very simple story of human sexual difference emerged: it is an anthropological fact that males and females look different from each other.

To name the conditions under which particular claims to difference emerge and are supported is not to deny that differences exist. It is instead to name those differences as products of human interventions rather than natural occurrences that humans simply record (Fausto-Sterling 2000). As Ousterhout's story of face-to-face sex determination suggests—and as most of our daily experiences attest—most of the time we are able to look at a person's face and place them into a sex category almost immediately. According to one American study, viewers correctly assess the facial sex of those they meet 96 percent of the time (Andreu and Mollineda 2008). These assessments are not based on universal and ahistorical biological truths about human bodies; they depend on who is looking and what they're looking for. For Candace, a middle-aged white person living in San Francisco, the unfortunate reality was that the people around whom she lived and worked recognized her as a man even when she felt she was a woman. It was this persistent and unwelcome recognition that brought her to Ousterhout's office.

If the maleness of Candace's skull was so pervasive that others saw it in spite of the feminine gender she cultivated, then Ousterhout needed to find a female skull that would move her just as reliably and predictably into the category of recognizable femaleness. He needed to move her into that 5 percent of the female population that appeared to the viewer to be almost certainly female because there were too many other things about Candace's body that signified maleness. The complexities of race- and age-based conceptions of femaleness and beauty are not confined to the dusty past of anthropological scholarship, of course. The ideas that informed early scholarship on sexual and racial difference continue to inform how women and men are defined and recognized every day. It was the everyday that Candace and Ousterhout wanted to change.

After consulting a number of sources,[8] Ousterhout determined that the forehead, nose, and chin were the primary sites in the facial skeleton that physical and forensic anthropologists examined to find sex-determining characteristics. Modifications to these bones were surgically safe and, he believed, could produce the most effective changes in gendered facial appearance. (For a graphic and textual description of these sites, see "Interlude: The Procedures.") The typological profile of the female skull—unmoored from its contextual and conditional relationships with the politics of race, age, and the scholarship in which it was produced—was a category that could travel.

Step Two: The Michigan Series and the Female Mean
Craniofacial sex entered the surgical realm as a pragmatic category. No longer a means of describing existing visible distinctions, it was meant to guide a plan for producing them. Equipped with a set of specific sites in the facial skeleton where sex differences were manifest—forehead, nose, and chin—Ousterhout next needed to quantify those differences in order to surgically produce them. If the forehead, nose, and chin are smaller in females, in what ways and proportions are they smaller, and how much smaller are they? Ousterhout's personal experience led him to a source that could answer those questions.

Prior to entering medical school at the University of Michigan, Ousterhout had earned a dental degree there. As a dental student he had worked as a research assistant on a long-term project measuring craniofacial growth in children and adolescents. The University of Michigan University School Growth Study (USGS) began studying children enrolled at the University School around 1930. Each year graduate students overseen by the Orthodontic Department collected dental casts of students in the first through twelfth grade, as well as radiographs of the lateral jaw and occlusal plane (the plane passing through the biting surfaces of the teeth). In 1953 the radiographs were replaced by lateral and posterior cephalograms (x-rays of the skull from profile and rear).

In 1974 the University of Michigan Center for Human Growth and Development published findings from the study in *An Atlas of Craniofacial Growth: Cephalometric Standards from the University School Growth Study* (Riolo et al. 1974). The "descriptive statistical information" in the *Atlas* represents measurements taken from eighty-three individuals (forty-seven males and thirty-six females) who attended the University School without interruption from the ages of six to sixteen. One of a wave of studies prompted by the Hoover administration's call to develop more research on "normal children," the USGS provided baseline information on the orthodontic implications of normal facial development.[9] According to James McNamara, the third author of the *Atlas*, the orthodontic interest in sexual dimorphism, then and now, is in estimating the age at which children's craniofacial bones stop growing. This information informs the timing and nature of orthodontic interventions. The fact that the USGS atlas produced a series of measurements describing the sexed morphology of normal faces was somewhat external to its primary function but played a significant role in the development and ongoing practice of facial feminization surgery.

Like all of the children included in the eleven major North American craniofacial growth research studies conducted in the early part of the twentieth century, the subjects of the USGS were identified as healthy and normally developing.[10] And all of them were white. Concerns about repeated exposure to radiation involved in annually x-raying children's heads halted these studies in the 1970s and has meant that no new longitudinal studies of this kind are being conducted today. As a result the research on these several groups of children constitute the "normal face" that continues to guide orthodontic practice.[11]

Ousterhout looked to the *Atlas* in order to quantify differences in the forehead, nose, and chin that his research in physical anthropology had identified. The *Atlas* provided the specificity of millimeters by which the "female skull"—an ostensibly neutral and universal form—could become a specific form: the female face. The data in this volume formed the basis for Ousterhout's measurement of "normal" male and female ranges of craniofacial structures. A copy of this book was sitting on or near his desk every day of my research in his office. Neon pink Post-It notes had marked particular pages for so long that their crumpled and exposed edges had faded to white. Though the numbers come from the *Atlas*, it has been many years since he's had to open the book to find them; they had long since been committed to memory.

The numbers that define the female face do not simply guide Ousterhout's surgical plan; they prescribe the values that must be accomplished in order to meet the burden of the female face; they are the metrics of facial sex change. Before beginning an operation, Ousterhout would place a patient's frontal and lateral cephalograms on the operating room light board. In the negative space of the cephalograms he stuck a Post-It that displayed three sets of numbers for each planned procedure: (1) the measurements he took of the patient's skull in the presurgical exam, (2) the USGS normal female range for each skeletal feature, and (3) the amount of reduction required to bring the patient into that range. Once the patient's skull had been measured, FFS was primarily a problem of subtraction.

In a presentation of his services to a group of attendees at a conference for trans- women and cross-dressers in 2010, Ousterhout explained how he used the USGS to plan patients' surgeries: "The University of Michigan had these series of cephalograms over fifty to sixty years. They've analyzed these, they trace them, and it's the source of a lot of records and some averages, extremes, standard deviations. We can come up with, based on your skull size, exactly where I want to put you to go from a male to a female. I do reserve some engineering, some aesthetic use of my thumb in the operating room—a little here, a little there—but I like to put things on pretty much a mathematical basis where you're going to be." Not only did the USGS numbers provide the exact definition of the female face that guided Ousterhout's surgical plan, but they did so in the authoritative language of mathematics. Leaning on claims to objective authority, Ousterhout safeguarded his claims to sexual difference from criticisms that often plague cosmetic surgeons: that the work they do is purely subjective, a reflection of shifting social norms and their own aesthetic tastes (see Gilman 1998). The figures in the *Atlas* allowed him to determine "exactly where . . . to put you to go from a male to a female." By invoking these numbers Ousterhout was able to identify female structure as a set of objective facts, a form he could reproduce with surgical precision.

Step Three: The Atkinson Library of Applied Anatomy

After conducting this foundational research on facial sex difference, Ousterhout had to learn to see skulls—these objects that had been the focus of his intensive study and notable career—in a new way. The final phase of his research took him to the Atkinson Library of Applied Anatomy, a collection of approximately 1,400 dry skulls housed at the Dugoni School of Dentistry at the University of the Pacific in San Francisco. Spencer R. Atkinson (1886–1970), a respected dentist and orthodontist, directed and oversaw the collection of skulls over a forty-five-year period beginning in 1919 (Dechant 2000).[12]

The aggressive practices and large number of collectors who contributed to the collection in its early years meant that there were no standards in terms of the information recorded about any particular skull. Many skulls lack the kinds of provenance that are typically used in such collections. Atkinson's colleagues traveling in Central and South America returned from their research trips with skulls about which they had no identifying information.[13] About some little more was known of the source than the word *Mexico* scrawled across the cranium in pencil. As a result of this missing and inconsistent provenance, the Atkinson Library is classified as a "mixed collection," one in which there is no distinction between individuals of different racial and ethnic groups. Sex is also difficult to discern in this type of collection. The library's curator, Dorothy Dechant, is careful to classify particular specimens as "probably" male or female, but she told me that she would be very hesitant to guarantee the sex of any particular skull. "The best we can say is 'probably,'" she stated.

Even if one did not know the sex of the deceased for certain, Dechant offered, one could line up a series of skulls to get a sense of the gradation in morphology that physical and forensic anthropologists typically use to distinguish sex. This is precisely what Ousterhout did: he arranged skulls on the table, masculine-looking to feminine-looking. However, when relative differences in morphology—"That one looks more masculine to me"—are read not as viewer impressions but as factual indicators of sex, the interdependence of race, sex, and age is, again, rendered invisible. In this kind of seriation exercise a skull that had been classifiable only in relation to others within its population group could now be independently evaluated against the observer's ideas of masculine and feminine aesthetics. Ousterhout found what he recognized to be typical male and female specimens in the Atkinson collection; they looked masculine and feminine to him, and so he asserted that the masculine skulls were male and the feminine skulls were female. The newly produced fact of their femaleness was used to underwrite his claim that he could surgically construct a distinctively *female* face. The gendered ideal of aesthetic femininity became the fact of female sex—not only descriptively but prescriptively as well. It was transformed from a look, an effect on the viewer, into a surgical plan.

Through this series of methodological interventions, authorized as they were by an abiding belief that the face can be understood and reproduced as a sexually dimorphic body part, Ousterhout succeeded in turning the "feminine type" of early physical anthropology into a contemporary prescription for surgical sex change. His formulation of the problem of facial feminization surgery has been long-lasting, and his contributions are widely recognized in this small field (Altman 2012; Becking et al. 2007; Bowman and Goldberg 2006; Davidson et al. 2000; Dempf and Eckertet 2010; Habal 1990; Hage et al. 1997b; Hoenig 2011; Morrison et al. 2016; Nouraei et al. 2007; Shams and Motamedi 2009; Spiegel 2011; Spiegel and Ainsworth 2010; Vázquez and Vila 2006).

The female face that emerged as a result of this research process was quite a specific one, though its claims to efficacy and utility as a sex-changing model relied upon—and continue to rely upon—its presentation as the form of naturalized, binary, and biologically determined craniofacial sex difference. The histories of racial categorization, of skull and cephalogram collecting, and of methodological choreography are absorbed by the surgical claim that opened this chapter: there are anthropological differences between male and female faces. The persistence and persuasion of this claim were supported by a commonsense view that human sexual difference is binary and essential. It was this view that structured Ousterhout's research and made it possible to interpret Candace's sense of alienation not simply as a phenomenological or social problem but as the logical result of a series of scientific facts. People didn't recognize her as a woman because she did not have a female face. But she could.

NUMBERS ARE CERTAIN, BUT THEY CHANGE

When Candace and her doctor approached Ousterhout in 1982 with the request that he rebuild her face, Ousterhout was treading on new territory but was guided by two principles that had shaped American trans- medicine for the prior thirty years. First, human bodies come in two mutually exclusive sexes: male and female. Thus research into sex difference involves using scientific methods to produce objective and actionable knowledge about natural bodily states. Second, sex difference is primarily a genital affair, and transsexuals are defined as such because they desire genital surgery. This assumption allowed Ousterhout to see facial surgery as auxiliary to and supportive of genital surgery. It also allowed him to operate on trans- women without a qualifying diagnosis because facial surgery didn't constitute the "irreversible" change of sex to which existing evaluation protocols controlled access. By operating on trans- women's faces, Ousterhout understood he was helping them to appear more like women, but it was genital surgery that made them women.

This set of assumptions, reflecting the political, institutional, and therapeutic logics of a particular time and place, would undergo significant change. Gaining momentum in the early 1990s, amid the rapidly changing queer politics and socioeconomic shifts in the San Francisco Bay Area, Ousterhout's practice would not remain tethered to this early model of transsexual medicine or the conceptualizations of sex and gender from which it came.

After Candace's operation word of her transformative facial surgery spread to other trans- women in San Francisco, and Ousterhout's FFS practice gradually began to grow. As he was committed to the scientifically derived sexual dimorphism that guided the development of FFS, the procedures he performed in the late 1980s and early 1990s aimed to give patients "normal" female faces. That is, he worked to bring their faces—mostly foreheads, noses, and chins—into the middle of the normal range presented in the USGS Atlas. In the mid-1990s, however, his relationship to those numbers and to the project of binary normalcy shifted in response to his patients' feedback. He explained this shift to the conference for trans- women and cross-dressers in 2010:

> [Early on] I knew what the average female had and what the average male had, and where the extremes are. It was interesting. In about 1992 I did a forehead II on [Paula], a lawyer from New York City.[14] My end point at that time was different. She looked very good, but she came back in about 1995 or '96, and she brought a lot of pictures of models. You couldn't make measurements on them, but what was obvious was that the [models'] foreheads were much further back than what I had been doing [for my patients].

By the time Paula returned to his office in the mid-1990s, Ousterhout's FFS practice was booming, facilitated by growing online networks and the massive flow of capital into the San Francisco Bay Area. By 1995 FFS constituted roughly 80 percent of his busy practice. The steady flow of paying FFS patients meant that in 1998 he was able to sever ties with the University of California and open his own practice. Ousterhout's was one of only a few private offices inside a hospital located in San Francisco's Castro District, one of the oldest and most well-known gay neighborhoods in the United States.

Attitudes about trans- people and approaches to trans- health and health care were undergoing significant shifts in the early 1990s, especially in San Francisco. Two influential activist groups, Transsexual Menace and Intersex Society of North America, were gaining influence in the city (Chase 1998). Important academic work in what would later be called gender theory was being published just across the Bay at UC Berkeley (Butler 1990, 1993; Laqueur 1990). Down the peninsula in Santa Cruz, Teresa de Lauretis introduced "queer theory" at a 1990 conference and institutionalized the term shortly thereafter (de Lauretis 1991). Outside the academy, Bay Area trans- activists were giving voice to visions of politics and embodiment that refused the paternalistic medical model in favor of a liberatory project premised on a self-determination that rejected pathologizing and assimilationist imperatives (see Bornstein 1994; Feinberg 1992; Stone [1991] 2006; Stryker 1994).

Activist, artistic, and academic shifts made their way into local public policy and medical practice. Responding to a citywide survey of the needs of transgender people and the exigencies of the ongoing HIV/AIDS crisis, the city of San Francisco created the country's first transgender public health program in 1993. Largely administered by one primary care clinic, the program abandoned the gatekeeping model used by the gender clinics that had dissolved a decade before. Instead of requiring a psychological diagnosis as the condition for receiving hormonal therapy, clinic staff adopted a consent-based model, allowing transgender patients to speak on their own behalf and directly request the health care resources they needed (Roebuck 2013).

Although the city's public health efforts were focused on high-risk transgender residents—a group that was generally underresourced and largely people of color—rather than the overwhelmingly white, resourced professionals that Ousterhout saw in his private surgical practice, local shifts in attitudes toward trans- people and institutional responses to their health care needs influenced Ousterhout's practice and informed his philosophy of care. The 1950s clinical model of transsexualism and its rigid program of treatment had been refracted by the emergence of *transgender*, a term whose relation to medicine remains complex and unsettled.[15] There was more than one way to understand and provide treatment for people who identified themselves as trans-, transsexual, or transgender. Treatment need not be focused on hormones and genital surgery, and the conditions of medical transition need not be directed by physicians' perceptions of narrowly defined binary sex difference alone. It was within this context that Ousterhout considered Paula's request to look more like the models in her magazine:

> She asked me if I could [operate on] her again. I did, and it made all the difference in the world. She was a female before; now she was an attractive female. It changed my whole end result. It changed my approach. Everything changed. It's given, as a result, a much more beautiful patient. . . . I'm more aggressive now than I was even two years ago. Most of my aggressiveness has been caused by patients who come back and say, "Can you take off a little more?" For example, the lower jaw. What I did in 1995 is quite different from what I do in 2010. I go much further. And I think my results are better because of that.

Although he considered Paula's original FFS a success, in that her face had been reconstructed within the ranges of the female norm and others regularly recognized her as a woman, she did not look like a model. "Average women are not beautiful," Ousterhout said to me plainly, "and average men are not handsome. I had been making average women; now I could make more beautiful women." "Normalcy," the goal of reconstructive surgery and the one that guided the essentialist philosophy of trans- medicine, had given way to another approach. By the mid-1990s, within a context of fee-for-service medicine in which trans- patients were newly authorized to articulate their own medical desires, Paula could ask to be something better than normal. She could join the ranks of millions of other Americans in the 1990s who were turning to surgery in order to realize their ideal selves.

While average femaleness had been guided by the middle of the USGS normal range, beauty was at its extremes. Ousterhout remained absolutely committed to the metrics of female form. After all, recognizability required representing forms that people expected. Though these numbers guided his practice until the day he retired in 2014, Paula's visit had convinced him that making patients "more beautiful" required removing more bone than was required to make them "female." They needed a narrower jaw, a more recessed forehead. Like the impetus for the initial development of the procedure, the drive to "go further" was spurred by patient request, but it also changed Ousterhout's perception of the goal of the procedures and the quality of his own work.

The skull measurements that had guided Ousterhout's early FFS work in the 1980s had, by the end of the 1990s, been modulated by the appealing ratios of female aesthetics. With the help of special new calipers developed by his son, Oliver, Ousterhout's version of "natural" sexual difference became more complicated. Incorporating the Greek ideal of the Golden Mean, his patients' feedback, the numbers from the USGS, and a will to "go further" than their norms described, Ousterhout's ideas about his patients' faces changed, and so did his ideas about what kind of changes FFS could enact. Following surgery his patients would *look like* women. And when others recognized them as such, they would *be* women.

HOW WILL I KNOW?

In April 2014 Ousterhout and I had dinner at a little French bistro in San Francisco's Pacific Heights neighborhood. As soon as we were seated the owner brought out a bottle of wine bearing Ousterhout's name on the label. The logo was a set of calipers for measuring the Golden Mean. Despite good reviews, wine sales were slow. It's a problem of marketing, he explained, of how to distinguish a good wine in a crowded field. Ousterhout planned to retire in a few months' time, and we sat, sipping the wine, discussing the progress of this book and reflecting on his career.

From the mid-1990s until his last day in the operating room, in August 2014, a typical week of work had included at least two FFS procedures. This amounted to nearly 1,700 FFS operations. His FFS patients had remained overwhelmingly white and unusually resourced. They were fighter pilots, accomplished athletes, Hollywood players, and decorated military officers. Fourteen of them had been nominated for a Nobel Prize. "Find me another group of seventeen hundred people who you could say that about," he bragged. He had seen patients from all over the world, as young as eighteen and as old as seventy-six. Though he had his share of critics (more on this later), he had also amassed legions of fans. Many patients showered him with praise, affirming that FFS had changed their life, making their deepest desires into their embodied reality.

Over his career Ousterhout became ever more convinced of how transformative facial reconstruction could be in the lives of trans- women. He explained its efficacy not by recounting the ratios that guided his surgical practice but by reproducing scenes of social life. He retold a favorite story about a trans- woman who lived two blocks from an elementary school. Even though she was recognized as female most of the time, he explained, every time she walked by the schoolyard the children would tease and taunt her, calling her a man and a drag queen. After her FFS the kids never teased her again. This story, like the imaginary scene of answering the door on a Saturday morning recounted in the introduction, shifts the location of sex out of the individual person's body and into acts of social recognition. It shifts sex from the essentialist and individualistic model that guided the emergence of transsexualism in the 1950s and its treatment through the 1970s into a model that stressed the social life of the body and the productive power of recognition. This new conceptualization of trans- therapeutics did not replace the old model; it took a place beside it, multiplying frameworks for what trans- people wanted from medicine and how surgeons could and should provide it.

"Can you believe that even today more people get genital surgery than facial feminization?" he asked, as I slid a beet across my plate. "It makes no sense to me." For him the shift from individual to social, from sex in bodily forms to sex enacted through recognition was so complete that it had become difficult to understand the project of medicosurgical transition any other way. For Ousterhout, and for the many hundreds of his surgical patients, the most important intervention in medical transition had nothing to do with genitals at all.

The Procedures

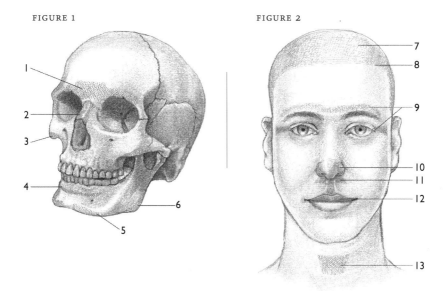

FIGURE 1

FIGURE 2

Ousterhout's research produced the following bone and soft tissue procedures as the means by which a male face could be feminized. These procedures are in use by contemporary FFS surgeons, though each has their own opinions about which procedures should be used in specific cases.

In general the procedures are aimed at removing or reducing particular bones and soft tissue features. The focus on reduction and removal is based on a fundamental assertion that male faces are, on the whole, larger and more robust than female faces. Whereas the modification of the facial

FIGURES 1 AND 2. Locations of the thirteen surgical procedures described in the text. Illustrations by Megan E. B. Foldenauer, PhD, CMI.

bones is often guided by metric norms, most soft tissue procedures are oriented toward an aesthetic ideal of youthful attractiveness. As one East Coast FFS surgeon explains it, femininity and attractiveness are synonyms.

Not every patient undergoes all of the procedures described here, though some certainly do. A patient whose surgery includes all of these procedures gets "the full face" or "the works." While one of the aims of this book is to trouble the claims to absolute difference that often animate FFS discourse, in the following descriptions I present the dichotomous distinctions that doctors use when characterizing the masculine features of patients' skulls and that patients often reproduce in describing their face and their hopes for transformation.

BONE PROCEDURES

1. BROW BOSSING AND FRONTAL SINUS: FFS surgeons assert that prominent brows and foreheads are definitive signs of maleness. Some reduction of the brow can be accomplished by grinding or burring down the thickness of the bones (known as bossing) just above the eyes. In other cases the anterior wall of the frontal sinus (the bone that lies just beneath the skin of the forehead) is sawed apart from the skull and set back into the sinus space, thereby reducing the distance the forehead protrudes beyond the plane of the patient's eyeball. Unroofing and recessing the frontal bone—what Ousterhout (1987) calls the Type III in his typology of forehead-altering techniques— is considered the most aggressive and invasive of all procedures involved in facial feminization surgery.

2. RHINOPLASTY: Rhinoplasty involves fracturing and resetting nasal bones as well as removing or reshaping cartilage. More radical bone fracturing and removal is required when frontal bone reconstruction (1) is performed. When the forehead is set back by unroofing the frontal sinus, the bones at the nasion (the depressed area between the eyes just superior to the bridge of the nose) must also be reduced in order to create the desired relationship between forehead and nose.

3. MALAR IMPLANTS: In order to produce the oval shape frequently associated with desirable femininity, implants may be placed over the malar (cheek) bones to make the cheeks fuller and softer.

4. GENIOPLASTY: Based on the claim that female chins are shorter than male chins (as measured from the top of the bottom teeth to the most inferior point of the chin), a wedge of bone can be removed from the chin to

reduce its overall height and width. Sections of bone can also slide forward (this is called a sliding genioplasty) in order to create a more pointed chin.

5. RESHAPING MENTAL PROTUBERANCE: Surgeons often argue that pointed chins are more feminine than square chins. In combination with the advancement of the inferior portion of the chin, the mental bone can be contoured to enhance this characteristic.

6. REDUCTION MANDIBULOPLASTY: Alterations of the mandible (jaw bone) focus on the squareness of the jaw that is often described as undesirably masculine. Squareness is attributed to two aspects of the mandible: its angle (whether the bone makes a sharply acute angle beneath the ear or a wide and obtuse angle) and mandibular flare (the extent to which the bony jaw extends out from the sides of the face). According to some FFS surgeons, the more acute the angle, the more masculine the jaw. Others argue that square jaws are not distinctly sexed characteristics. Through burring and excision, bone can be removed in order to reduce undesirable squareness and flaring. Portions of the masseter muscle can also be removed in this effort.

SOFT TISSUE PROCEDURES

7. SCALP ADVANCEMENT: By severing the tissue that connects the scalp to the skull, the scalp may be brought forward toward the face. This procedure helps to make the forehead appear smaller and can sometimes compensate for a receding hairline. Some patients also use topical creams or hair implants or transplants to manage hair loss. When the scalp is advanced and the hairline reshaped, the eyebrows can be raised on the forehead. This is intended to open and brighten the eyes and eliminate wrinkles associated with aging. All of these are performed through the coronal incision (from ear to ear just behind the hairline) required to alter the bony contours of the forehead (item 1).[1]

8. HAIRLINE RESHAPING: In addition to bringing the hair-bearing scalp forward, the hairline itself can be reshaped. In this procedure a hairline can be rounded out to reduce (if not eliminate) temporal "male pattern" baldness caused by a byproduct of testosterone.

9. EYEBROW RAISING, CROW'S FEET REDUCTION, FOREHEAD LIFT: Eyebrow raising, crow's feet reduction, and forehead lift are performed at the site of the coronal incision after the bone work on the forehead has been completed (item 1). When tissue is excised during scalp advancement (item

7) or hairline reshaping (item 8), the position of the eyebrows may be raised higher on the forehead. The appearance of the eyebrows is also changed as a result of modifications to the bones of the brow and forehead beneath them. During this procedure surgeons have access to the internal muscles of the forehead and may choose to perform a perforation of those muscles; this procedure is typically referred to as a brow lift.

10. RHINOPLASTY: Structures of cartilage give shape to the tip of the nose. After the bone modifications have been made (item 2), the cartilage can be reshaped in order to achieve a more feminine nose. Feminizing a nose generally means reducing the size of its tip and directing its tip either straight ahead or slightly upturned.

11. UPPER LIP SHORTENING: According to the surgeons with whom I worked, males have a longer upper lip (as measured between the bottom of the nose and the upper ridge of the upper lip) than do females. This distinction can be seen most easily by observing how much of the upper teeth are visible when a person's mouth is slightly open, called "tooth show." The length of the upper lip can be reduced by excising tissue just beneath the nose, raising the upper lip toward the nose, and applying sutures in the crease just at the base of the nose. This also results in increasing the amount of vermillion visible in the upper lip, thereby giving it a plumped appearance.

12. LIP AUGMENTATION: Lips can be augmented by a variety of procedures, including by injecting pharmaceutical products (such as Botox and Restylane) or fat taken from other sites in the patient's body. More permanent augmentation can be achieved by placing some of the tissue excised during the scalp advancement (item 7) into the tissue on the underside of the upper lip. Lip augmentation techniques vary according to surgeon preference.

13. REDUCTION OF THE THYROID CARTILAGE: The thyroid cartilage, or Adam's apple, is considered a definitive indicator of maleness. Thyroid cartilage removal is commonly referred to as a tracheal shave (or "trach shave") despite the fact that the trachea is not altered, nor is anything shaved. Though a relatively simple procedure, thyroid cartilage reduction carries significant risks. If a surgeon removes more tissue than necessary, permanent damage to the vocal chords may occur. Thyroid cartilage reduction can be performed through an incision just below the point of the chin or sometimes through an incision in the middle of the throat directly above the cartilage itself.

2 · Femininity in the Clinic

Coordination into singularity doesn't depend on the possibility
to refer to a preexisting object. It is a task. This is what designing
treatment entails. —Annemarie Mol, *The Body Multiple*, 2002

To develop plans for surgical interventions, surgeons apply the general principles of their knowledge and training to the specific body of their patient. In the case of FFS, the surgeon begins by assessing the gender signifiers of a patient's face. Which characteristics make this face masculine? What must be changed in order for it to be feminine? Given my technical abilities and strengths, how will I go about making those changes? Surgeons answer these questions in relation to their own sense of how facial masculinity and femininity are defined and often in consultation with their patients' visions and desires. Like all forms of surgical sex reassignment, facial feminization surgery materializes ideas about bodily sex difference into sets of technical practices. In order to operate, surgeons must establish an end goal, an aim to guide their interventions and in reference to which an outcome can be considered good or bad, successful or not. When FFS surgeons design a plan for intervention, they materialize their understandings of what women look like. At the same time, when they argue alongside their patients that

FFS is central to—and sometimes itself instantiates—a patient's physical transition, they also enact a therapeutic logic, an understanding of the ends toward which trans- surgery works and a claim to how particular technical interventions can be used to reach those ends. While FFS physically transforms a patient's face, the efficacy of the procedure is determined not by the postoperative shape of the face per se but by the responses that her face elicits from others. As such, when FFS works it makes many things: a new face is one, and a new claim to the therapeutic ends of trans- surgery is another.

Ousterhout's original development of FFS was guided by principles of binary sex difference and his understandings of the "wrong body" to "right body" aim of transsexual transition. Though over time his metrics of facial sex difference moved from the center of the "normal" range to its idealized extremes, he remained committed to the objective and mathematically derived distinctions of sexual difference through the end of his career. He believed that in order to be recognized as a woman, a trans- woman's masculine face must be made to adhere to the metrics of normal female form. But Ousterhout's method of defining male and female faces and designing surgical plans for their transformation is not the only approach to FFS. His was neither the only means for enacting woman nor, as a result, the only way of understanding what trans- women want from FFS.

In this chapter I analyze two initial patient consultations, one in Ousterhout's office and one in the office of Joel Beck, a cosmetic surgeon. Both of the surgeons and both of their patients share a common goal for FFS: that after surgery the patients will be recognized as women. Despite their common goal, the two surgeons have different ideas about how to realize this result. Committed to the recognitive power of binary normalcy, Ousterhout recommended that his patient's face be brought into the extreme ranges of metrically normal femaleness. Pursuing an individualized therapy of self-optimization, Beck encouraged his patient to collaborate in designing a plan that would increase her "sex appeal."

More than surgeons' individual or stylistic differences, differences between these consultations represent contrasting and coexisting paradigms of trans- therapeutics that have emerged in American trans- medicine over the past thirty years. Ousterhout and Beck have different ideas about what women look like and about the reasons for which trans- women seek surgical services and the ends toward which those services should be attuned. Alongside the lasting midcentury model of illness and cure that guides the practice of surgeons like Ousterhout who are committed to making trans-women "normal" is a growing therapeutic philosophy adopted by those like Beck that frames surgery for trans- people as a means to individual authenticity and self-optimization. In such a framing, trans- people join the ranks of millions of other Americans who turn to surgery not because they're sick or need treatment but because they can and believe they should become the best and most authentic selves they can be. This version of health—the open-ended, self-directed, aspirational kind—is the kind that market medicine favors. And it was a kind of trans- medicine that had not been possible thirty years before.

ENACTING WOMAN IN THE CLINIC

Knowing what a woman looks like is not easy, and, as it turns out, establishing an internally coherent model of trans- therapeutics is not either. Annemarie Mol (2002:vii) has argued that it is through practices of intervention that medicine "enacts the objects of its concern and treatment." Rather than imagining that transsexualism or gender dysphoria (or whatever qualifying diagnosis one might choose) is a stable condition that exists in the world and to which doctors respond, Mol's approach begins from actions themselves. Resisting a collapse into sameness by attending to the differences of practice, Mol argues that as an object of medical intervention, the body is more than one thing at once, and so are the conditions that organize clinicians' interventions. The best way to understand this multiplicity is to watch how it gets done.

The diagnostic entity once known as transsexualism (in the third edition of the American Psychiatric Association's *Diagnostic and Statistical Manual of Mental Disorders, DSM-III*), later gender identity disorder (*DSM-IV*), and now gender dysphoria (*DSM-5*) may be one of the very best examples of how medicine multiply enacts its objects of intervention. There has never been a clinical consensus about the origin or nature of the issue for which trans- people seek medical intervention.[1] To the extent that there is an increasingly accepted standard of care, that care centrally involves the coordination of disparate forms of knowledge, expertise, and evidence. Psychotherapists hear stories of gender difference and produce a mental health diagnosis. Medical doctors respond to that diagnosis by prescribing hormones. Surgeons respond further by rebuilding bodily structures. Letters, recommendations, and diagnostic codes coordinate the actions of these practitioners, who may share a recognized currency of "the same" diagnosis (First 2010), but in practical terms the "conditions" they treat have little in common. Childhood stories that pique psychotherapists' interest are irrelevant to physicians who read blood panels when determining hormone prescriptions. Those same blood panels are irrelevant to surgeons who do their work with burrs and sutures. Following Mol, it is clear that trans- therapeutics work differently in each of these places; it is only the claim to diagnostic cohesion that makes them appear to hang together, to be responding to and helping to constitute the same thing. (For an early description of the coordination work in the German context, see Hirschauer 1998.)[2]

The benefit of understanding diseases and diagnoses as produced through forms of clinical practice is that one can see how relationships between a diagnostic entity like transsexualism or gender dysphoria or the female face and its forms of treatment are negotiated and renegotiated in the course of everyday life. In consultation rooms and operating rooms surgeons' therapeutic logics are enacted differently than are psychotherapists' and medical doctors'; one surgeon might also enact trans- therapeutics differently from another surgeon.

MEET DR. BECK

Twenty miles south of San Francisco, in the suburb of San Mateo, Joel Beck was actively working to grow his facial feminization surgery practice. Beck began his career in cosmetic surgery as the junior partner of a small private clinic. When we first met in 2010 he had taken over management of the partnership, and by the time I returned to visit in 2014 he was running the practice on his own. As a cosmetic plastic surgeon he specialized in surgical and skin care treatments that aimed to help patients "enhance their natural beauty." From liposuction and tummy tucks (offered in combination in the "Mommy Makeover") to rhinoplasty and facelift, the practice was dedicated to rejuvenation and beautification.

Beck told me that in 2005 his senior partner suggested that he think about adding facial feminization surgery to his list of services. Having completed a fellowship in craniofacial surgery during his medical education, Beck had some experience with the bone work that differentiates FFS from the facial surgery he typically performed in his practice. Though he considered himself technically capable of performing FFS procedures, Beck was reluctant at first. At the time he did not know anything about transpeople and was worried that the stigma attached to them would attach to him by association (Goffman 1963:30). Several years later, however, he was grateful that he had followed his senior partner's advice. At the time of this writing payments from FFS constituted roughly 30 percent of his annual revenue. "Thank god I started doing FFS," he said, "because there are a million plastic surgeons now, or people who want to be plastic surgeons." Beck was working to grow his business with trans- patients, looking for ways to increase his presence in trans- social media and drive traffic to his FFS website. He had recently established a formal collaboration with an endocrinologist and prominent genital sex-reassignment surgeon in an effort to develop what he hoped would become "a hub of transgender medicine."

The fact that Beck's work with trans- patients began in 2005 not as a response to a patient request or as the result of his personal interest but as a strategy for financial success attests to the massive changes in trans-medicine that had occurred since the early 1990s. No longer a marginal or derided specialty, performing surgery for trans- patients was a smart business decision for a surgeon otherwise competing in the mainstream cosmetic surgery market. If the demand for FFS were not so high in the Bay Area, Beck likely would have found it difficult to establish a reputation for the practice. As it was, it took him only a few years to grow his business through word of mouth. He did this, in part, by casting his approach to FFS in direct contrast to Ousterhout's. Beck's difference of approach did not stem from a definition of the female face that contrasted with the one Ousterhout originally established. Instead he disagreed with the idea that creating "normal" females ought to be the goal of FFS.

Beck understood FFS as responding to a particular set of *desires* more than a particular pathology or a grouping of measurable physical characteristics. He saw his trans- patients' desire to appear more feminine as one that was shared by virtually all of the women who visited his office. As such, Beck did not identify his FFS patients as people with distinctly male faces; instead he saw them as women who were unfortunately unattractive in a predictable set of ways that could be improved with particular bone and soft tissue procedures, electrolysis, and skin care regimens. Divorced from the pathological legacy of transsexualism, in which gendered identity and sexed anatomy were said to exist in mismatched binary pairs, FFS was for Beck simply a means to the kind of self-optimization and aspirational beauty sought by all of his patients.

Beck came to trans- medicine long after activists had begun working to separate sex and gender difference from psychopathology. More than ten years had passed between the disappearance of transsexualism from the DSM in 1994 and when the first trans- identified patient walked into his office. He was not contending with the legacy of the old university gender clinics and had no stake in the political battles over pathology or diagnosis. As a cosmetic surgeon he was accustomed to working outside the purview of insurance coverage and did not concern himself with whether or how FFS might be regarded by insurance companies any differently from the other elective procedures he performed. He felt no need to investigate clinical histories or ongoing struggles over definitions of gender as an "ordered" or "disordered" thing. Beck did not attend meetings of the World Professional Association for Transgender Health, nor did he plan to do so in the future. He did not linger at trans- conferences any longer than was required to give his own presentations and meet with potential clients.

Although Beck and Ousterhout ostensibly shared a common aim for FFS, the different moments in which they entered the practice of trans- surgery and their different clinical orientations to surgery itself meant that how they understood and materialized woman in their patients' faces were quite distinct.

AGAINST PATHOLOGY

When American university-based gender clinics closed in the early 1980s, trans- specific endocrine and surgical services moved into private practice. The strict diagnosis and access protocols that university clinics had employed were gradually replaced by more patient-centered treatment models that reflected the competition and individualism of market medicine (Bolin 1988; Meyerowitz 2002). In the process the "wrong body" illness narrative of transsexualism that had been produced and reproduced in university clinics was fractured and complicated. Taking up newly emerging narratives of gender difference, activists argued that the will to pathologize and medicalize particular forms of gendered being and embodiment was itself indicative of a pervasive *social* pathology. They were not sick; it was a sick society that labeled them so. Adopting the name "transgenderists," a word that had been coined by the American Virginia Prince in the late 1980s, activists took cues from civil rights, feminist, and gay and lesbian movements as they worked to end discrimination against those who did not fit within the narrow limits of contemporary gender norms. Gordene MacKenzie's (1994) *Transgen-*

der Nation made use of anthropological texts to argue that gender variation was a cross-cultural and transhistorical phenomenon that was arbitrarily structured and unjustly pathologized in American medicine.[3] "By rejecting medical definitions and categorizations that stigmatize them as having a 'psychological disorder,'" MacKenzie wrote, "transsexuals and transgenderists can shift the emphasis from a personal 'disorder' to a cultural 'disorder.' This shift forms the nucleus of the Gender Movement" (6).

Like many of her contemporaries, rather than seeing transgenderism as a problem to be cured or overcome, MacKenzie believed it was an identity category with transformative potential. The activist Holly Boswell (1997:56) wrote, "The newly emerging paradigm of gender will lead to a potent activation of healthy and renewable alternative gender expression. Yes, this shift is new. Never before have we had so many options, yet chosen to manifest—despite our culture—our *true selves*." Such narratives figured transgender people as bravely confronting, in part by physically manifesting, the contradictions of an oppressive gender system. If the either/or of the binary system enforced division and hierarchy, the both/neither of the transgender figure was staged by some as a personally bold and symbolically potent refusal of its terms.

While some early 1990s trans- activists rejected the paradigm of disorder and paternalistic control in favor of celebrating the transformative potential of gender transgression (Bornstein 1994; Feinberg 1992; Stone [1991] 2006; Stryker 1994), others opposed diagnostic pathologies on the grounds that they denied individuals the fundamental right to self-determination. Taking up a claim to bodily autonomy likened to a woman's right to abortion, Nancy Nangeroni (1997) argued that the paternalistic and pathologizing model of midcentury psychology denied trans- people the right to control their own body. "For any person other than myself to exert final authority over decisions of what to do with this physical body is a violation of my personal autonomy," she wrote (351).[4] Rather than arguing against surgical intervention in favor of gender transgression, as Prince and MacKenzie did, Nangeroni wanted to refigure the place of surgery in trans- medicine. Those who shared Nangeroni's position felt that access to body-altering surgery should not depend upon pathologizing diagnoses or be controlled by powerful surgeons. Instead they used rhetorics of self-determination to assert that people should decide for themselves when and what kind of surgery to have. Emphasizing American values of autonomy and independence, an individually articulated desire for surgery was itself a legitimate reason to have surgery and to compel a surgeon to perform it.[5] "The vesting of authority in the individual," Nangeroni wrote, "will promote diversity while supporting the growth of personal dignity" (350). For her the act of denouncing the paternalism and pathology inherent in diagnostic and access protocols and instead granting autonomy and self-determination to trans- people would render its own form of affirmative therapy, apart from whatever surgery might accomplish.

The ideal of the "healthy" "individual" who realizes her "true self" through the exercise of "personal autonomy" suited the America of the late twentieth century (Edmonds 2009; Gilman 1998; Haiken 1997; Serlin 2004). Increasingly organized by the ideals of personal responsibility and market-oriented solutions to personal and social problems, and galvanized by a queer political push-back against Reagan-era policies of weakened social programs and devastating silence on the impact of HIV/AIDS on sexual minority communities, a new space for "transgender" people began to emerge.[6]

At the same time enormous increases in the number and size of American medical schools between 1965 and 1980 flooded the market with new physicians, a surfeit that drove doctors into ever narrower medical specialization (Starr 1982). In 1982 the U.S. Supreme Court lifted a long-standing ban that had prevented physicians from marketing their services directly to patients (*Goldfarb v. Virginia State Bar*). Now free to compete and eager to avoid the oversight and massive paperwork required from the expanding insurance industry, more and more doctors began performing elective procedures for which patients paid on a fee-for-service basis. Between 1970 and 1996 the number of physicians who designated their area of specialty as plastic surgery increased by 269 percent (Sullivan 2001:74).

By the end of the dynamic 1990s the midcentury model of sex and gender by which the diagnosis, characterization, and treatment paradigm of transsexualism was first established had undergone radical shifts. No longer relying on justification from a contested discourse of pathology and treatment, desires for sex- and gender-transforming surgery found a new claim to medical legitimacy in the growing discourse of medicine as a means of authenticity and self-optimization (Davis 2003b; Gagné and McGaughey 2002).

The surgical consultations I present exemplify two coexisting and sometimes antagonistic paradigms of trans- therapeutics that continue to structure trans- medicine in America. The first one, represented by Ousterhout, adheres to the idea that trans- people seek surgery to resolve a "wrong body" problem. In this paradigm the distress caused by living in the wrong body can be mitigated by surgically intervening to create the "right" one. Right bodies are defined by the desirable normalcy of anatomical forms and tend to be figured in a binary model in which one sexed body can be altered into the form of *the* other. It is in the instantiation of bodily rightness that dysphoric distress is relieved and by which trans- medicine is good medicine.

In the second treatment paradigm, represented by Beck, the aim of trans- medicine is to make manifest the patient's sense of self that, as a result of particular bodily forms, has been invisible or obscured. In this therapeutic paradigm the trans- patient's distress is due to the fact that their individual and "true self" is not recognizable in their current bodily state. Hormonal and surgical interventions are used to manifest their internal sense of self, which may or may not correspond to a binary model of sex. This model of trans- therapeutics is patient- rather than clinician-centric and therefore allows a greater range of bodily forms to result from the processes of transition. Emerging in the 1990s as a result of efforts to depathologize gender difference and to dislodge the "incorrigible proposition" that human bodies come in two mutually exclusive sexes (Kessler and McKenna 1978), this paradigm foregrounds self-expression and self-actualization as modalities of treatment and their measures of wellness.

These different trans- therapeutic models shaped how surgeons understood their patients' goals, and thus how they assessed patients' faces and which forms of intervention they recommended. In recommending particular surgical plans, Ousterhout and Beck enacted the category of woman in ways that reflected their perspectives on the treatment they were providing and that also had material effects in their patients' flesh and bone.

TRACY'S CONSULTATION

From his private office in a large hospital in San Francisco's Castro District, Ousterhout could walk to the surgical wing, where operating rooms and surgical recovery rooms were located, in less than a minute. His was one of only a few private clinical offices in the main hospital. Visitors entered the hospital through the wide sliding Emergency Room doors and followed a corridor to his office. When I entered the exam room, a new patient named Tracy was seated in the reclining exam chair, nervously scraping at her black nail polish. The etching on the wall behind her of a naked reclining woman rendered in bronze and silver tones stood in garish contrast to Tracy's jet-black hair and black crushed-velvet tunic. From the wall-mounted rack in front of her—and so behind Ousterhout when he conducted her exam—Fergie from the Black Eyed Peas stared out from her enviable place on the cover of *Allure* magazine. For months she looked on as Ousterhout assessed the undesirably masculine faces of his patients, baring her midriff in an unceasing smolder.

Ousterhout urged Tracy to keep her seat as I introduced myself and shook her hand.[7] As usual he began the appointment with a few minutes of friendly conversation, inquiring about Tracy's Canadian hometown and sharing a story of his travels there some twenty years before. He used these first moments to establish a rapport with new patients, who were frequently very nervous—and in some cases could best be described as star-struck.

Ousterhout then moved on to questions about Tracy's medical history: her height, weight, medications, prior surgeries, and so on. When Tracy stated that she was actively losing weight and would like to get down to 180 pounds, Ousterhout made his first recommendation of the appointment. "I'd like to see you down to 160," he said. "The best results I see—not surgically but in terms of overall femininity—are in patients who get down to a female weight for their height. When you get down to 180, just keep on going." While unrelated to the craniofacial consultation under way, Ousterhout's recommendation on "overall femininity" signaled his definition of FFS as part of a larger project of corporal feminization that took its guidance from the metrics of bodily norms and the ideals of desirable beauty. Ousterhout did not ask Tracy what her goals were for surgery; he simply pulled a flexible white ruler from his coat pocket, rolled his stool up to her chair, and got to work.

After taking a series of measurements from Tracy's face and from the cephalogram (profile x-ray) she had brought with her, Ousterhout recommended a number of surgical procedures intended to bring her into the ideal part of the "normal" female range that he had identified. He recommended unroofing her frontal sinus in order to set her forehead back 8 millimeters; cutting out the flaring of her mandible (the squareness at the back of her jaw); burring down the ridge of bone beneath her bottom teeth; cutting out an 8 millimeter wedge of bone to reduce the height of her chin; advancing her hairline 1.5 centimeters; raising her upper lip 4–5 millimeters; reducing the dorsum (bridge) of her nose; reducing the projection (tip) of her nose; reducing the prominence of the glabella (where her nose meets with her forehead [frontal] bone); and removing her thyroid cartilage (Adam's apple).

Ousterhout explained the recommendations by invoking the metrics of the female norm as narrowed by the idealized feminine aesthetics that he had honed over the years. For example, when determining how much to set back Tracy's forehead, he said, "I could take you back eight millimeters. The fifteen millimeters you currently are minus eight equals seven millimeters. That is where I want you. If you had an X chromosome rather than the Y you were born with, that is where you'd be. You got this [indicating her brow prominence] when you were fourteen, fifteen, sixteen years old." In reference to her chin, he explained, "I measured from the top of your bottom teeth to the end of the bone, and that is fifty millimeters. That is average for a male of your height. I want to take out eight millimeters of chin height." Of her hairline he said, "Right now the distance from your brow to your hairline is seven centimeters. I want five and a half centimeters. The average male has a distance there of five-eighths of an inch longer than the average female. This is the case in sixteen-year-old males, even before they've experienced hair loss."

Recommendations that did not come with specific numbers were explained in reference to a general characterization of how males and females are differently built. For example, he described using an oscillating saw to "get rid of the bowing that males have in the mandible that females don't have." Sometimes Ousterhout's own face stood in as the exemplar of male form. When explaining how the ridge below her bottom teeth could be removed, Ousterhout placed Tracy's index finger on the side of his face. "Feel my teeth?" he asked. He pressed her finger into his cheek and moved it back and forth so she could feel the texture of the bone below his bottom teeth. "Feel that ridge? That is what we take away." When explaining why he recommended raising her upper lip 4 or 5 millimeters, he said, "Now your upper lip has a vertical height of two and a half centimeters and drops two to three millimeters below your upper teeth. If you look at me when I talk, you don't see my upper teeth unless I smile." He smiled at her. "You see?" In these instances Ousterhout's face became the model by which he could establish points of common masculinity between his face and hers. His face was that of a normal male; unfortunately so was Tracy's. With these forms of demonstration Ousterhout made Tracy's maleness into an observable thing, transforming her sense of gendered disconnection and nonbelonging into a materially real property that she could see and feel (Miravel 2008). Using palpation and measurement, Ousterhout enacted Tracy's maleness in order to articulate the potential of her future femaleness.[8]

What is clear from this consultation, and the many others I observed, is that while Ousterhout's approach to the definition of the female face had changed somewhat over his thirty years of FFS practice, it was still a definition oriented to an essential and binary model of sex difference. In this model male and female faces are discrete and mutually exclusive structures that reflect distinctions in the sexed body traceable down to the chromosomes. The claim that setting Tracy's forehead back 8 millimeters would give her the forehead she would have had if she had been born with XX instead of XY chromosomes not only called up the normative authority of the University School Growth Study; it also laid claim to a broad and totalizing bodily history, linking Tracy's bones in the exam room to the image in her cephalogram, the hormones that had acted on her body thirty years earlier, and the chromosomes that were, in this telling, responsible for it all. Ousterhout believed that in order for Tracy to be recognized as female, her face must look as though it had never experienced the changes effected by testosterone during puberty. His approach was recuperative of the prepubescent face Tracy once had, and in that way it would also be redemptive of the life she longed to have. Biological stories do more than describe biologies.

For Ousterhout, Tracy's case was quite straightforward. The sexually binary model of facial forms dictated that if a trans- woman had a body that was measurably normal for males—which he found that most did—then a particular set of procedures must be performed to make her face normally female. Tracy would have been free to disagree with Ousterhout's diagnosis and recommended interventions of course. She could have said that despite his definition of a normal female chin, she wanted to leave her chin as it was or to alter it in some less invasive way. But binary models are incompatible with half-measures. "Less is not more," he stated. "We've had over the years not more than four or five patients probably, who came in and said, 'You were going to set my forehead back eight millimeters, just go four.' Or 'You want my chin to go up six, just do three.' 'You're going to move it forward eight, just go four.' Fine. I'll do that for you, but you're not going to be happy. Every one of them has come back and said, 'Go ahead, fix it,' because they still look masculine. You've got to go there. It's crazy, but you've got to do all these things." In this telling "normally" female is the only thing that is not recognizably masculine. While normal may be a range within which one can move, the effectiveness of its instantiation is not up for negotiation. If normalcy is the goal—and the model that treats FFS as reconstructive surgery for a measurable form of sexual difference says that it is—then Ousterhout is its arbiter.

LEANNE'S CONSULTATION

Beck's practice was located in an office park and shared a building with accountants, attorneys, and dental offices. It also included the Ambulatory Surgical Clinic, where he performed most of his operations. In the waiting room a leather couch and several armchairs were arranged around a coffee table covered in fashion magazines. The dominant feature of the room was a mirror-backed, top-lit curio cabinet featuring branded cosmetic products such as Juviderm and Botox. The occasional pouty stillness of the faces of the young women who staffed the reception desk made it clear that they were sometime users of the products they helped to sell.

When Beck invited me in to observe the consultation, Leanne was seated and waiting. Leanne was one of the few patients I encountered who arrived for an FFS consultation in what was referred to as "man mode" or "male mode." She had taken the opportunity to visit Beck's office while traveling through town on business and looked every bit the businessman: closely cut blond hair graying at the temples, a crisply pressed pale blue shirt, gray trousers, and black oxford shoes. Beck quickly waved away Leanne's apology for having arrived at the office dressed this way. He opened the conversation in his usual way, by asking her how she had heard about him and his practice. This positioned Leanne as a consumer who had shopped around and identified Beck as a service provider eager to grow his practice. After a bit of small talk Beck began the exam not by taking a medical history but by prompting a personal conversation. "Tell me about yourself," he said, "about your transition."

Leanne spoke in a measured voice:

I began dealing with my gender issues at fifty, when my wife and I became empty nesters. I've already been cleared for hormones, but I'm waiting to take them until after my daughter's wedding in a few months. I'm a manager—I mean, that's what I do for a living, but that's also who I am. I like to have everything figured out before I start. That's why I'm here. I don't really know how hormones will affect me and what changes they might make to my face, but I do know that my face is the most important thing to me. I can do things with clothes, but I can't hide my face.

Beck perched motionless on his stool as she spoke. "Making changes to your face can make you more feminine-appearing," he affirmed. A practiced interviewer, he allowed her silences to go unfilled.

I know that if I proceed with this my marriage will be over, and I understand that. My wife didn't really sign up for all this, and I can't force her to feel better about it. I'm here because I want to manage my expectations; I need to know realistically where I might end up instead of going forward with all of this and then finding out that you can't do what I think you can do. I don't want someone to give me all of the classic female things. I was interested in talking to you because you said that you work *with* features, not totally remake them. It's not a clean slate. Given the face that I have, I want to know what to expect. Right now I don't look like a woman; I look like a man in a wig. I haven't gone out much; I only wear women's clothes when I go to counseling. But when I go out I worry about my face. I want to look like me, like how I feel. You know?

Beck did not verbally respond to any of Leanne's personal and emotional disclosures; he simply began the physical examination by taking a handheld mirror from the drawer behind him. He handed it to her. She looked at her face in the mirror as he spoke.

"We'll start at the top and work our way down," he said. "These are only suggestions to let you know what's possible and how I think of things. We think of the face in three sections: forehead, midface, and lower face. One of the most feminizing effects happens in the forehead. We can move the hairline forward. But bone work is required to make a feminine skull." Beck retrieved a model skull from the counter behind him and used his index finger to show Leanne how the frontal bone could be reduced. "By burring down this area [above the eyes] instead of removing the bone, we can retain the angle from your forehead to your nose. Patients with 'the works' often look worked on. That is not what I want to give you. When you lose the natural transition from the forehead to the nose you don't look good as a man or a woman." Such recommendations both communicated Beck's surgical approach and argued for their superiority over the kinds of recommendations that Leanne would likely hear from surgeons like Ousterhout, whose reputation for radical forehead reconstruction was well known in the field. Leanne had specifically said that she did not want "all of the classic female things," an indication that she was familiar with Ousterhout's approach and wanted something different from Beck.

Still Beck felt that Leanne's forehead should be reduced. Rather than unroofing the sinus, he recommended burring down the bone. He ran the pad of his thumb across the ridge above Leanne's left eye as she looked at her face in the mirror. "Reducing this will give you the feminine appearance. It gives you sex appeal. That's the approach we're going for." After emphasizing what he did not what to do—give her "the works" that would make her look "worked on"—Beck articulated that his approach was to give Leanne "sex appeal." This category is implicitly marked as feminine, but it was not one that relied on fixed ideas about biological femaleness. Burring down the bony prominences above her eyes was one part of his plan, but it also involved aspects of her face that were not coded as male. "Now, when I'm in doing the forehead contouring," he continued, "I can remove some frown muscle, which would be nice for you." Removing the frown muscle is a procedure typically performed as part of a brow lift or forehead lift. While there is nothing distinctively male about frown lines, their removal is undertaken to create the youthful appearance associated with feminine beauty. Leanne's sex appeal would be ensured not only by reducing her bone but by restoring her youth.

Beck explained the value of shortening her upper lip in the same way. "The upper lip could be shortened. That is really common in feminization surgery. It'll be like when you were younger." He pressed the wooden handle of a cotton swab just beneath Leanne's nose, causing her upper lip to rise on the surface of her teeth and allowing more tooth to show. Rather than referring to an external model of normalcy by which Leanne might understand her long upper lip as a normal but undesirably male characteristic, Beck explained it as an unfortunate part of aging. By pressing the swab under her nose, he was able to show her how her face could be changed to be more aesthetically desirable—more youthful and sexy—not necessarily more essentially female.

Beck's departure from the morphology of female craniofacial norms was most pronounced in his recommendation not to alter Leanne's jaw: "In terms of the jaw, I would leave it alone." Leanne was surprised to hear this. She put the mirror on her lap and turned to face him. "Really?" she asked. "Beautiful women have a strong jaw line," he explained. While delivering a presentation at a conference for trans-women, Beck told his audience that many famous surgeons are now putting mandibular angle implants into female patients. He was saying that many women who want to be beautiful—and the surgeons who work to make them so—want to have precisely the kind of wide jaw that many trans-women already had. Jaw tapering "is a disservice" that is often performed by those with "a systematic approach" to FFS, he explained. "For you," he told Leanne, "brow lift, cheek implants possibly to give you some more fullness in the midface, and nose for sure. If you'd like to see what this would look like, we can image you and give you a better idea of what I am talking about."

Beck led Leanne to a small, dimly lit room adjacent to the exam room. I looked over Beck's shoulder as he took digital photos of Leanne's face and uploaded them into a laptop.

"I try to do things with imaging that I can do during surgery so that it's not unrealistic," he said. "One thing would be to decrease projection of your nose. Come over here and I'll show you what I mean." Leanne sat beside Beck in front of the computer. Using a stylus and trackpad, Beck circled the areas that he could reduce in the frontal bossing, orbital bossing, and nose projection. As he moved the stylus from left to right across the trackpad, the nose, forehead, and orbital bossing all reduced in unison. As he moved back to the left, they "grew" back to their original size. Leanne sat expressionless as she watched her face grow and shrink, grow and shrink.

After a few seconds during which she did not speak, Beck stepped in. "I'm kind of limited in what I can show here," he said. "I mean, you have to imagine what it would look like once your facial hair is gone. You've also got some skin damage that you should really work on. I'd say the most important thing you can do for yourself between now and any surgery would be to start a skin care regimen. Work on that sun damage and some of the brown areas, the wrinkles around the eyes." As he indicated these problem areas on the computerized image of her face, he offered to make an appointment for her to see an esthetician. "I really do think that is really important. You know, beautiful women have beautiful skin." With this intervention Beck tried to reframe the reasons Leanne seemed unhappy with the images he showed her. It wasn't a limitation of the proposed surgeries, he suggested, so much as it was difficult for her to see past the familiar surface of her own face. Her skin was damaged and blotchy. She had unwanted facial hair and wrinkles around her eyes. If youthful beauty was the goal, these things would spoil it regardless of the architecture of her face. Leanne agreed.

She said the years she'd spent in Arizona had done a lot of damage, and she looked mournful about a lifetime of choices that had resulted in the wrinkles and spotted skin that Beck helped her to see as a significant and unwanted part of her gendered appearance. This narration of facial difference was a significant departure from the one that framed the distinctly sexed face as an inevitable effect of sex chromosomes.

"Here are some other patients I've operated on," he said. "Maybe these will give you a better idea of the changes I'm talking about." He opened a computer file with several pre- and post-op images of his patients. He clicked through the images, describing the procedures he'd performed. "Here you can see I did the nose. . . . Here you can see the reduced bossing; that really opens up the eyes. . . . Here you can see the difference that a brow lift really makes. She looks great." Beck tried to narrate the images so that Leanne could see them positively. To be convincing the images would have to appear to be transformative for the people depicted in them and Leanne would need to see herself as potentially transformed in the same ways. It wasn't working.

"These people look much more feminine than what I see when we look at me," she said. "I have my wig with me. Can I put it on and have you take the pictures again?" Beck appeared reluctant, but he agreed to take a new profile photo. She crouched down and pulled a reddish-brown shag-cut wig out of her briefcase. It was disheveled and needed brushing. While the mirror had been the technology of visualization in the exam room, in the tiny imaging room the camera and computer had taken its place. Leanne could not see herself until she was pictured on the computer screen, waiting to be modified. Not on quite straight, the wig screamed its contrast with her shirt and tie. One of the qualities that made the wig desirable to her—that it obscured her forehead and brow—also made it problematic for the photo shoot.

"Could you pull your hair back so I can see your forehead?" Beck asked. Leanne brushed back her bangs and Beck took the photo. She resumed her seat beside him at the computer. Her disappointment with the new image was evident. Beck reiterated the importance of starting a skin care regimen and beginning electrolysis on her face. "I think those changes could make a big difference for you," he said. "Let's go talk to my office manager, Jasmine. She can give you a better idea about prices, and we can look at some more images." I stayed behind as they left the room and went into Jasmine's office. "Do you think I could ever look this good?" I heard Leanne ask as she looked at the curated collection of before-and-after photos in the album. "I'm worried about going through all of this and looking as ridiculous as I do now." "I think we can do really great things for you," Beck reassured her. Then he left her to consider his recommendations and to discuss the matter of payment.

Beck's assessment of Leanne's face and his recommendations for surgical intervention were not based on a biological or anatomical claim to essential differences between male and female faces. He did not narrate Leanne's concerns with her appearance as deriving from her unfortunately male characteristics. Instead he read her masculinity as (fixable!) misfortunes of aging, unattractiveness, and inadequate self-care. As such, hers was the same kind of masculinity that haunts the abject outside of feminine beauty for many who seek it. Though he articulated the aims of FFS in the same way that Ousterhout did, Beck's different definition of woman and therefore of the properties that instantiate or spoil it meant that his surgical practices enact these things differently as well. At stake in these distinctions are the very definitions of what it means to be sexed, to be gendered, and to be transgendered. By this I mean that if Beck's different approach to woman also works for his patients, then the fact of its efficacy effectively recasts his understanding of what brought his patients to the office in the first place: they didn't need to be normal females in order to be recognized as women; they did not need to reject one "wrong body" for another "right" one; they needed to be beautiful individuals. The effect and its methods differently cast the cause.

IF BEAUTY IS THE END, FEMALENESS MAY NOT BE THE MEANS

"Jennifer Aniston has an enlarged lower face and a strong chin," Beck explained to a conference audience who had gathered to hear his talk "Aesthetic Subtlety with Feminization Surgery." He and Ousterhout both gave talks during the conference weekend, and many participants attended both presentations in order to compare approaches. Their ability to attend both sessions was a point of contention for Beck. He had coveted Ousterhout's prime Saturday midmorning slot but had to settle for a less popular Friday afternoon time. These kinds of prioritizations were an uphill battle for him as he tried to build his reputation.

Gwyneth Paltrow's "forehead is enlarged," he said. Angelina Jolie "has an enlarged forehead, a recessed hairline almost. She has a broad jaw. She has a protruding chin. Yet she's considered to be one of the most beautiful women in the United States." As he spoke these women's larger-than-life faces beamed from the projector screen behind him. We audience members were invited to see these women—whom we'd already seen countless times—as people who had characteristics that were typically considered masculine but who were undeniably beautiful. Masculine features, we learned, were not always manly ones, and they weren't always at odds with beauty.

Naming a nonsexed ideal of beauty as the goal of FFS enabled Beck to work outside of the prescribed ranges of the osteologically female and instead make subjective alterations in pursuit of a desired aesthetic. He was after a look rather than a structure. Or, as he told Leanne, he was going for sex appeal. He felt that it was this look—the effect of the feminine rather than the structure of the female—that patients ultimately wanted from FFS. He believed his patients would be recognized as women when they were seen as youthfully beautiful.

"People are often attractive because they DON'T conform to statistical norms," Beck assured prospective patients on his FFS website. "Statistically, women have more pointed chins than men, but this does not mean that pointed chins are prettier. They are just more common. Facial feminization surgery should not be used to 'normalize' features that contribute to beauty." These passages define femininity not as the property of femaleness but as the effect of beauty. They both reject the statistically normal female and rely on the stability of that norm in order to identify beauty as its exception. It was not the accuracy of Ousterhout's measurements that Beck was contesting; it was the utility of their application. "Commonness" is not what someone should aspire to when "prettiness" is an option, he suggested. The collapsing of biological femaleness with desirable beauty that had silently facilitated Ousterhout's development of FFS is here made explicit. Common is ordinary—even statistically average—not beautiful.

In other conference rooms other FFS surgeons were making their own pitches about how to define the *feminization* in facial feminization surgery. Some leaned more toward Ousterhout's empirical approach, drawing on osteological models and measurements, and others more toward Beck's. The latter group drew heavily on celebrity photographs, supplying patients with examples of facial form that were also aspirational. I have seen Michelle Pfeiffer, Grace Kelly, Jodie Foster, and Renée Zellweger offered as examples of female facial form, and George Clooney, Brad Pitt, Burt Lancaster, and Matthew McConaughey as their male counterparts. Some surgeons claimed that feminization required removing the angular jaw. Other surgeons swore against it. Dr. Morris, a plastic surgeon better known among prospective trans- surgical patients for his work on genital transformation procedures but who had recently begun to perform FFS, argued adamantly, "Guys like Ousterhout want to chop off your jaw, and I think that's terrible. The jaw has nothing to do with femininity or masculinity." In such conference presentations, ostensibly meant to inform patients but also clearly used as a marketing opportunity,[9] surgeons' first task was to define the female face (Talley 2014). This kind of definitional work did not play such a prominent role in the genital surgery presentations given just down the hall. There the issue was more about technique. But the main work done in the FFS talks was rhetorical: in order to advocate a surgical approach, surgeons began by making a case for what men and women look like and what must be done to move a person from one category to the other.

Just as Ousterhout's "normal" female face was based on measurements taken from young white women, the celebrity models that Beck and other FFS surgeons used to demonstrate feminine beauty were also always white. Although surgeons tended to dismiss my questions about the effect of such models on viewers—one insisting, "They're just examples. Nobody thinks we're trying to make people look white"—patients sometimes voiced other responses. Gretchen planned to have FFS with Ousterhout and then sometime later travel to Thailand for genital surgery. The Thai surgeon could perform FFS, but Gretchen said, "He seems to be doing a lot of Asian faces. So I'm a little bit afraid of asking an Asian guy to do work on me that he usually does on Asian faces." A patient named Krista also planned to travel to Thailand for genital surgery but found the prospect of getting FFS done there "really iffy." Krista also worried about an "Asian specialist" working on her face. While these patients didn't consider doctor-patient racial similarity to be important in reconstructing genitals, facial feminization required a kind of in-group sight in which patient and surgeon are matched pairs (see Lam 2005; Pitts 2006).[10]

Beck's goal of individual beautification was ostensibly both unraced and not reducible to sex-specific characteristics. "The wide mandible is attractive in men or women regardless of its statistical prevalence between the sexes," he explained. He demonstrated this point in his presentation slide show by projecting images of wide-jawed and beautiful (and white) Brad

Pitt and Johnny Depp. While a square jaw may have made physical anthropologists unsure about the sex (or race) of a particular skull and may therefore be a principal site of Ousterhout's interventions, in Beck's estimation—and Morris's too—such an unusual feature was an asset whose uniqueness defined the beautiful. For Beck single characteristics of the face could not be defined as male or female in isolation. Sometimes femininity is quintessentially female, as Ousterhout defined it, and sometimes it is not.

Using this approach in the clinic Beck allowed Leanne to articulate her own goals for surgery. Because her consultation began with the disclosure of intimate emotional information, the examination that followed became a response to that information. She wanted Beck to "work with" her features and to make changes that would help her "fit in." The pull of this desire was bound up in her intimate relationships with her daughter and her wife; their needs became part of the story she told about why she had come to his office and why she may or may not come back. Brought into the consultation through the use of visualizing software, Leanne was faced with more than agreeing or disagreeing with Beck's recommendations; she had been shown a possible future and was left to decide if it was one she could embrace.[11]

WHAT'S AT STAKE IN A MODEL
OF TRANS- THERAPEUTICS?

In order to ask after the efficacy of FFS—whether it "works"—one first has to decide what it would mean for FFS to work and how such a thing could be determined. Both of the surgeons and all of the patients I talked with agreed that the efficacy of FFS depended on whether other people recognized the postoperative patient as a woman. Of course this recognition does not happen in the operating room or in the surgeon's office; it happens sometime and somewhere in the future, in some interaction or, preferably, *every single* interaction for the rest of a patient's life. Enacting a therapeutic paradigm of normalization or individual self-actualization means staking a claim to the kinds of changes that must occur in order for the patient to be recognized as normal or self-actualized. That claim locks etiology and efficacy into place; it implicates a particular understanding of the issue that FFS is meant to address (fixing a wrong body or making an authentic self visible) and a particular kind of health (normalcy or optimization) that will be achieved when it does so. These therapeutic logics guide surgeons' work, and (prospective) patients use them to make sense of their embodied experience before and after their surgical encounters.

Ousterhout wanted to make Tracy normal, and Beck wanted to give Leanne sex appeal. Their recommendations took the form of distinct surgical procedures and would involve particular risks, time away from work, protracted healing, and a significant fee. Both aimed to arrive at a corporal and recognizable femininity that would significantly change their patients' lives, but they did not share a definition of femininity, nor therefore did they agree on the surgical means required to instantiate it. Since Ousterhout's feminization was guided by an ideal of binary biological femaleness, when his procedures worked he saw Tracy's case as treatable through the instantiation of binary normal forms. Because Beck's feminization was guided by an ideal of aesthetic distinction, when his procedures worked he saw Leanne's case as treatable through personalized interventions that allowed her unique self to be rendered visible on the surface of her body.

When both of their divergent approaches work—when both result in patients being recognized by others as women—the effect is that two coexisting trans- therapeutics are enacted. These surgical enactments help to frame FFS patients' sense of what was surgically possible and helped them to imagine and to plan for their own bodily futures. They gave substance to medically mediated models of sex, gender, and transgender, defining each of these terms and their relations to each other as a condition for their material interventions.

MAKING PLANS

Neither Tracy nor Leanne ended up scheduling surgery immediately after their consultations. Both had more thinking to do. Tracy had been saving money for three years before she decided to visit Ousterhout in person. She had found out about him online and over a great many hours of research had learned about the kinds of changes FFS made possible. She knew about other surgeons and how they described the work they did. She planned to pursue a comparative consultation by sending photographs of herself to another surgeon, but she'd spent the little money she had for in-person consultations to see Ousterhout. Tracy found his explanations compelling. Her hope for surgery was that it would result in "fewer stares." She spoke in a diminutive voice. "Yeah, fewer stares. Fewer stares. I just want people to walk by. I guess you could say that I'm out [as trans-] because I don't keep [my trans- identity] a secret. Because I *can't* keep it a secret. Sometimes I wonder if I could keep it a secret if my attitude would be different. But that's irrelevant. I can't keep it a secret. Not now at least. I don't think I want to keep it a secret. But at the same time, I don't want to scare small children." After this last sentence she began to laugh uncomfortably. When I began to laugh with her, she stopped me short. "Don't laugh," she said flatly. "I do." My smile disappeared and I wilted in my seat.

Tracy was confronting a series of agonizing choices, a calculus of risks and rewards that did not fit together easily. When she walked down the street, people stared and children recoiled. This wounded her deeply. Ousterhout's promise was that when his numbers were instantiated in her face, she would be normal—well, a different normal anyway. Physical normalcy was an embodied promise of invisibility: she would simply be a normal woman, no staring or scaring required. Tracy wanted people to walk by, to see her as a woman like any other and thus not really see her at all. After years of hiding herself under long hair and draped clothing, she wanted to be ordinary. Becoming normal would come at the cost of tens of thousands of dollars, of the physical pain of major surgery, and the emotional cost of pinning her hopes for well-being to an unknown future face that could change her identity. Or not. Ousterhout was certain, but how could she be?

Leanne headed straight for the airport after her consultation with Beck. Her visit to his office had been a brief detour in a business and family life in which she was rarely able to engage her identity as Leanne. Having scheduled the appointment largely because she happened to be in town, she was not yet ready to make decisions about surgery. "I would live [as a woman] full time if I were passable," she explained, "but I don't know if I can do it otherwise." Leanne would not seek medicosurgical interventions to manifest her sense of herself as a woman unless she could do so sufficiently well. Though she wanted to be "passable," she also wanted to look the way she felt. She wanted Beck to forgo the "classic female things" in favor of an approach that rendered her internal self visible to others. Her desire was not only to blend in but to bring a sense of her individual identity to the surface of her body. "I don't want to have a bunch of surgery and end up looking weird," she told me after her discussion with Jasmine. "Would that be any better? I just don't know."

Though Leanne had not experienced the same kinds of exclusion and derision that Tracy had, she feared such interactions; she did not want to look as "ridiculous" as she felt. She had gone out "dressed" enough to know that people recognized her as trans-, and the feeling of conspicuousness frightened her. If Leanne's concern was that her male body didn't "look like her," then occupying a body that had been surgically altered but still didn't look like her was not really a solution to that concern. If she could not reasonably expect to be recognized and accepted as a woman *and as herself*, Leanne didn't know whether transitioning would be worth all that it would cost her. For her, transitioning only to look "like a guy in a wig" didn't really amount to transitioning at all. "What would be the point of that?" she asked me resignedly.

Treatment strategies and surgical techniques help to enact forms of post-operative womanhood and particular iterations of sex, gender, and transgender to which it corresponds, but these clinical tools do not work alone. The controversial and turbulent past of American trans- medicine shapes clinical interactions, giving a distinctive tenor to the acts of care produced between a patient, her surgeon, and his staff. The history and politics of trans- medicine remain central to enactments of surgical care. But first a conference field trip.

Celebrate!

Celebrate! is an annual conference for cross-dressers and trans- women that has been held in the same rural town since 1990. There are only a small handful of these conferences in the United States each year, and many people attended as many of them as they could. In addition to informative presentations, conferences were important places for folks to build community, to feel accepted and seen as they were.

Throughout the weekend as I attended workshops, talks, and social events, shopping excursions and fashion shows, I chatted with people about FFS and surgical interventions more generally. With the exception of Rene, who was attending her first trans- conference and was generally blown away by everything she saw, everyone I spoke with had an opinion about facial feminization surgery.

I met Molly before the "Cross-Dressing 101" workshop. When I asked her about FFS she responded quickly, "I like everything I've got, just how it is." Molly was consistently recognized as male, but that didn't bother her. Cross-dressing was an occasional practice that she really enjoyed, but she had no interest in transitioning or changing her body in any permanent way. She compromised with her wife about little changes: Molly shaved her chest and body hair during the winter months and let it grow out for the summer swimsuit season.

Just because people knew about FFS did not necessarily mean they were interested in undergoing the procedure. During the second night of the conference I joined the official evening event at a town bar hosting a locally famous cover band that specialized in pop songs from the 1980s and 1990s. Their big conference draw, though, was that all the band members were cross-dressers. The small bar was packed with an amiable mix of town residents and conference attendees, making it a people-watching event for all tastes. In between beers and sweaty dances I struck up conversations with trans- women who were leaning against the wall or seated at the bar, watching the scene. "Yeah, sure, faces are a big deal," Gina told me, shouting against the thrum of the music. "But the real tell is the hairline. You can have a beautiful face, but if you're bald, no one is buying you as a woman." I heard these kinds of rejoinders a lot. Another person told me the voice is the real key. What good is a pretty face with a baritone voice? Another said hands were most important. Another said shoulders. For these trans-women FFS might have been desirable, but facial surgery alone would not have made the difference between being recognized as women or not. For them that line was located somewhere else on the body. Even beautiful faces would not have been enough.

Sophia knew two people who had had FFS. She said "they really do look much more feminine" and that her friends considered FFS to be the most important thing they'd done in their entire lives. While she acknowledged the transformative power of FFS, there were two reasons she was not interested in it for herself. "I'm six foot three," she said, "and there is nothing I can do about that." Like the women I met at the bar, Sophia understood other characteristics of her body—in her case, her height—were more determinative of her perceived sex than was her face. Changing her face on top of her tall frame would have been ineffectual. "More important," she said, "I have this." She picked up the silver walker she used to help her get around. "Once people see the walker, they really don't look at anything else about me." Dressed in a skirt and blouse, wearing a shag-cut gray wig, and leaning against a walker, Sophia was recognized as a woman most of the time. In part, she explained, because people don't look so closely at old women or disabled women. These characteristics of her body already deflected the scrutinizing and sexualizing gaze that subject many other women to viewers' judgment. Other folks sharing our conversation considered Sophia's walker to be an ingenious strategy. They joked that she had a great prop and that a walker was far cheaper than an operation. Sophia played along. "Oh yeah, I've got it all worked out," she said with a smile.

Femininity is an ongoing achievement. For some people facial surgery was the first and most important thing to do in order to achieve the femininity they desired. For others it was learning to move differently, or returning over and over again for electrolysis to remove beard and chest hair, or finding an elusive strappy sandal in the right size. Some other challenge comes next for everyone and becomes the thing that is standing in the way of the embodiment they desire. This is the way of sex and gender.

For many folks at the conference the first necessary step in pursuing femininity was learning to see it. Ousterhout and Beck offered two among many forms of expertise on that subject as they explained to attendees what made their face masculine and what must be done in order to achieve the femininity they desired. The surgeons' talks were well attended by hopeful viewers who wanted the characteristics of their face explained as plainly as the presenter for "Cross-Dressing 101" had explained how to hold a handbag. And while some audience members listened intently, scribbled in their notebooks, and booked individual consultations for later in the day, other rooms at the conference were teeming with people whose future would not include FFS. Elese said she was too old. Mona was happy just as she was, thank you very much. Jackie couldn't afford it. Shana just didn't have the stomach for it. These folks wanted something else from medicine or wanted nothing at all.

3 · Cutting as Caring

Thank you Dr. Ousterhout. Now I can "face" the future.
—On a plaque from a grateful patient

Treatment strategies and surgical techniques help to materialize forms of postoperative womanhood, and their approaches implicate distinct understandings of the reasons why and toward what ends trans- women seek surgical interventions. Treatment strategies and surgical techniques are not the only tools of trans- medicine, however; they unfold in a clinical setting whose palpable emotional charge is as central to the practice of FFS as any surgical cut. The controversial and turbulent history of American trans- medicine shapes ongoing clinical interactions and gives a distinctive tenor to the acts of care produced between a patient, her surgeon, and his staff. Examining the affective dynamic of the clinical space shows how the history and ethics of trans- medicine remain central to ongoing relationships between surgeons and their patients and significantly impact how, as what, and for whom trans- medicine works.

American medicine has been and largely remains neglectful of and punitive to trans- people,[1] making the intimacy between surgeons and patients a crucial part of the surgical dynamic and centrally shaping how trans- therapeutics are enacted. The practice of FFS is shaped by what Milligan and Power (2010) call a "geography of care" within which surgeons and patients make sense of their roles and relationships to each other, the histories to which they are heir, and the regulatory mechanisms of law, market, and medicine that structure their dynamics. It is within a distinctly American geography of care that acts of surgical precision emerge as practices of what I term *restitutive intimacy*. Surgical intimacy is restitutive when acts of surgical care in the present are, at the same time, also framed as compensatory responses for mistreatment and neglect in the past. Expressly shaped by the troubled past of inadequate and predatory surgical interventions for trans- people and formulating itself in contrast to it, the success of FFS depends upon its characterization as an act of compassion, an intimacy whose enactment of self-actualization is also a form of restitution, of justice done. Sustaining this characterization requires constant maintenance. In order to understand medicine as *part* of the lived reality of trans- subjectivity rather than a practice that *responds* to it, restitutive intimacy must be seen not as extraneous to the practice of trans- surgical care, but as a vital element of it. Deeply affective connections—of gratitude, loyalty, vulnerability, and compassion—between patients, surgeons, and their staff make it possible for FFS to do the work that it does.

GOOD CARE FROM BAD

Stories of trans- people's mistreatment by doctors and other caregivers are legion. In November 2011 the *Miami Herald* broke a story about a "fake doctor" who had injected cement, silicone, and other industrial materials into the hips and buttocks of a local trans- woman in order to give her "the derriere of her dreams."[2] In the following weeks more victims came forward, including one who reported that this "fake doctor," Oneal Ron Morris, had injected similar materials into her face two years before. The results were disastrous, producing, as one Miami news station put it, "acutely lumpy cheeks, [a] misshapen chin and a ballooning upper lip."[3] This client explained that she had heard about Morris through word of mouth in the trans- community and that she initially sought Morris's services because she could not afford a licensed surgeon. She told reporters, "It becomes so dire that you want to match your outside with your inside that you're willing to roll the dice and take your chances. As a transgender person, you're thinking, 'Oh, my God, I can start to look like I want to look like and I don't have to spend a lot of money.'"

A 2011 *New York Times* article focused on the popularity and risk associated with unlicensed injectors, or "pumpers."[4] A trans-woman, S., who had self-administered silicone injections to feminize her face

> sees herself as helping the women she injects. "I try to help the girls because they want to look feminine," she said, caressing the contours of her face to demonstrate. Her overly plump apple cheeks and smooth pink lips are telltale signs of the silicone injections she has given herself over the years. They dwarf her small, sculpted nose and dark brown eyes, which gleam under the thin eyebrows she carefully draws on. "I try to guide them because the majority of these girls are young," she continued. "They come to me with holes, dimples; they don't have no cheeks, and their face is long."

After three or four injection sessions, S. explained, she can help her clients achieve the looks they desire. Her methods may be unorthodox and considered by physicians to be extremely dangerous, but she claims that her results speak for themselves. On the day the *Times* reporter visited her home office, thirteen people were waiting to be "pumped."[5]

Stories of dangerous, backroom medical interventions for trans-women are not new. Take the notorious case of John Ronald Brown, an American surgeon who, by his estimate, performed genital sex-reassignment surgeries on six hundred trans-women from the 1970s until his imprisonment in 1998 (Meyerowitz 2002:271–72).[6] John "Butcher" or "Table Top" Brown, so known for his reported willingness to perform surgeries anywhere on anyone who could pay (Denny 1992; Whitlock 2001), was eventually convicted of murder after a patient-requested leg amputation went bad.[7] Brown was reported to be a disheveled and otherwise strange man, sometimes eating and drinking during surgeries performed at his bare-bones Tijuana clinic. The journalist Paul Ciotti recounts details of the story:

> Despite Brown's flaws, says Cheree [a former patient], there was a reason why so many [trans-] "girls" went to him—"He gives you a vagina at a fair price." Whereas with other doctors you had to take hormones, wait up to six years, live as a woman, undergo psychological evaluations and then pay $12,000 to $20,000 or more, with Brown it was good old-fashioned capitalistic cash-and-carry. Anyone, says

Cheree, could raise the necessary $2,000 or $3,000 Brown used to charge (in the '80s) by turning "a couple of tricks." The word would go out that Brown was coming to town. "He'd shoot silicone anywhere you wanted it. For $200 he'd do breast surgery. For $500 he'd do cheeks, breasts and hips. After injections you had to lie flat on your back for three days so the silicone wouldn't go anywhere. He plugged the holes with Krazy Glue."[8]

At the end of the long and bizarre 1998 murder trial during which judge and jury were made to view gory homemade videos of surgical procedures, there was little doubt of Brown's guilt. Sheldon Sherman, Brown's exasperated defense attorney, argued that though Brown may have been a terrible surgeon whose carelessness had indeed resulted in a patient's death, he ought to be lauded for his willingness to treat transsexuals. According to Ciotti, "Sherman chose to portray Brown as a brave and caring man who tended to a segment of society no one cared about. 'No one else would deal with transsexuals,' he said in his closing argument. 'John Brown said, "I'll deal with them." Did he do this for money? No. He did it because he cared.'"

Milligan and Power (2010) use the term "geography of care" to name the ways in which specifics of place shape the conditions of the care that is given there—and, in this case, what comes to count as "care" at all. It is because American trans- medicine has been so neglectful, punitive, and exclusionary of those without financial resources that the services of illicit practitioners have been and remain so desirable. It was within this history and geography of care that Brown's attorney could construe acts of brutality as "caring" about "a segment of society that no one cared about." Brown claimed to care for transsexuals because he was willing to operate (even disastrously) on poor trans- women when their lack of money and the stigmas against them meant that others would not.

Of course these terrible outcomes are not the only ones that emerge from the geography of American trans- medical care. At the same time that marginalized and fee-for-service medicine has created a large group of transpeople who are excluded from surgical services, there is another group who can and do pay out of pocket for the services of a small number of surgical specialists who have spent their entire careers treating trans- patients. This was the group of patients I met in Ousterhout's and Beck's offices. They were doctors, lawyers, entrepreneurs, professors, military officers, and career civil servants with generous pensions. The surgeons this group of trans- patients saw made a claim to care opposite to Brown's. These surgeons cared because they didn't let stigma against trans- women keep them from offering the very best surgical treatment money could buy.

The daily dynamic within the FFS clinic was saturated with the past and present of poor care, limited options, and the reality that money really could get some patients something that many other trans- women longed for. So it was that patients often interpreted a surgeon's skills as deeply intimate and exceptional practices of restitutive justice and compassion. It was from this same dynamic that surgeons gained a sense of reward and gratitude from patients that centrally motivated their work; the care they gave was reciprocated. These dynamics are not extraneous to the enactment of FFS; they are essential to its functioning. They shape the relationship between surgeons and patients, determining how, as what, and for whom FFS can work.

Ousterhout's and Beck's reputations as good surgeons reflected the work they did in the operating room and, crucially, the way they did it. Their entire clinical practices—from the marketing efforts aimed at attracting patients to the follow-up care provided long after surgery—was attuned to crafting an ethical and affective dynamic that attended specifically to the hostility and turbulence of American trans- medicine and constituted itself in contrast to it. This contrastive effort emphasized an intimacy between surgeons and their patients that foregrounded the emotional ties between them while diminishing the financial ties. In this intimate space of goodness, surgeons' acts of technical precision were framed as acts of beneficent "compassion," "friendship," and "goodwill" among a trans- population for which such goodwill is consistently framed as a scarcity. Patients' personal experiences of being treated poorly by other doctors—and store clerks, and DMV employees, and family members, and strangers on the street—and their fears that the vulnerable space of the clinic would turn into a place of hostility made doctors' compassion incredibly valuable. It was a critical facet of the care that doctors and their staff provided in the enactment and materialization of surgical womanhood.

MARKETING BENEFICENCE

American surgeons frequently market services to trans- patients by reproducing key features and rhetorical structures of trans- narratives. In so doing they present themselves as more than technicians. In contrast to imagined other doctors who would deny and stigmatize trans- women's desire for body modification, these surgeons portray themselves as operating for the reasons and toward the aims that trans- women articulate for themselves; they take on trans- women's desires as their own.

Dr. Lubbock, a midwestern FFS surgeon, promises his trans- women patients, "The face and body that you *should* have been born with is well within your grasp." Accompanied by the image of a hopeful and pensive young white woman, this text from his website reproduces a central theme in trans- self-narratives. Jay Prosser (1998:83) has discussed the recuperative language of "what should have been" as a trope in transsexual self-narratives that invokes a form of nostalgia, "a literal and figurative re-membering." Such language reimagines the history of the body as a body that existed in the desired form from the very beginning, one that never required surgeries, sutures, and the injection or ingestion of hormones. Surgeons' communication of technical practice carries strong affective messages about desirable bodily forms and helps to cultivate prospective patients' relationships to those forms (Braun 2009). This is not just a promise of bodily improvement; it is a promise of bodily reintegration, a making right.

An East Coast FFS surgeon, Dr. Gold, emphasizes the affective work that FFS accomplishes over and above the techniques involved in its performance. He defines FFS as procedures that provide patients with "the face they should have been born with" and uses the term "gender confirming facial surgery," seeing his goal as being to create facial features that support patients' "true gender."[9] Gold defines FFS as confirmation rather than transformation and invokes the language of "true gender" that many transpeople use to describe their own sense of sexed and gendered self as being more true and authentic than the way others have seen them.

Beck maintained two separate websites: one for his mainstream aesthetic surgical practice and one for his facial feminization practice. As opposed to the mainstream site's sleek images in black, bronze, and copper, his facial feminization site performed "feminine" in a more stereotypical way. Formatted in shades of violet and purple, its menu options were marked by brightly colored daisies. The words "beginning of a vision," "transition to femininity," and "a holistic approach" ran across the screen. The site included links to the pages of an affiliated endocrinologist, a preeminent American genital sex-reassignment surgeon, and several trans- conferences across the United States. There were also links to nonmedical gender services such as a femininity coaches, shopping assistants, and a business that made custom corsets for atypical feminine bodies.

Maintaining a trans- specific website helped Beck to produce a feeling of exclusivity and privacy for potential trans- patients and portrayed him as singularly committed to helping them realize their feminine selves. From the color schemes to the grand statements about patients' life experiences, this site was one way Beck demonstrated his special care for trans- women: he not only knew *what* trans- clients wanted from a surgical result; he also knew *why* they want it. Presenting this kind of care was central to the market by which prospective patients found the few surgeons who specialized in the procedures they desired. The dedicated FFS site also enacted a separation between his service for trans- patients and his services for others.

The care work done by these surgeons is not a one-way dynamic. Patients reciprocated surgeons' care by treating them as exceptional people with the power to do exceptional things. Patients' gratitude and effusive praise were important to Ousterhout and Beck, who reminded me over and over again that the reason they loved to work with trans- patients is because those patients made them feel so good.

GRATITUDE

While Ousterhout did not set out with the intention to work with trans- patients, he had made a concerted effort to make FFS the focus of his private practice since he began performing the procedures in the early 1980s. He explained his decision in very simple terms: his trans- patients loved him, and it felt good. Their sincere and effusive gratitude was extremely rewarding. "Transgender patients are more grateful for what I do for them than the parents of kids whose skulls I've rebuilt," he said. This is no small statement. Earlier in his career Ousterhout had directed the center for craniofacial anomalies at the University of California's San Francisco hospital. His patients included infants and children with devastating deformations of the face and skull, many of which required a series of major surgeries to correct. While these correctives were always undertaken with the aim of producing a "normal" appearance, they frequently also enabled essential functions such as breathing and swallowing. As a parent myself, I was especially struck by this measure of gratitude: even more than the parents of these children, trans- women were *grateful* for the surgeries he performed.

"Before, it was the parents of the children who loved me. Now it is the patients themselves," he said. Their love and gratitude mattered to him. Patients told him all the time that he changed their lives, that he saved their lives. They hugged him and shook his hand and thanked him. Many remained fiercely loyal.

To one former patient named Jill, Ousterhout was nothing less than a hero. After her procedure nearly ten years earlier, the two had become friends. In her testimonial foreword to Ousterhout's book on FFS she wrote, "There is nobody like him, and, most likely, there never will be. He cannot be replaced. He has no peers." Jill knew without a doubt that Ousterhout had profoundly changed her life. "I will be his strongest proponent," she told me resolutely. "I always tell him, if he's got somebody coming down on him, I'll take care of him. I can take care of myself and I will take care of him."

Because of its contested history and the current opt-in mode of treatment, in which doctors must decide they want to specialize in procedures for trans- people because they are not trained to do so in formal medical education (Obedin-Maliver et al. 2011), a doctor's willingness to treat trans- patients is often interpreted by patients and explained by doctors as a humanistic or compassionate act rather than one to which they are professionally obligated. Interpreting surgical procedures as acts of care and intimacy creates a powerful affective dynamic between patient and surgeon. This connection runs both ways.

Beck frequently reminded me that he preferred working with trans- patients because their sincere gratitude was so fulfilling. "If FFS could be my whole practice that would be great," he said. "I love these patients. They're nice. They're respectful. They're happy to have someone pay attention to them. They care about taking care of themselves, and they're thankful. It's nice to have someone who appreciates you."

The frequency with which surgeons mentioned their trans- patients' gratitude made it clear that this characteristic set them apart from other patients. Beck's remarks implied contrasts to other patients who are not nice, not respectful, and not thankful. His comment that "they're happy to have someone pay attention to them" also underscored the affective component of their relationship. These patients, who have come to expect poor or hostile care, appreciate his positive attention.

Trans- patients' appreciation took many forms, including direct statements of praise to the doctor as well as letters, cards, and gifts for the surgeon and his staff. Patients often expressed their thanks immediately following their procedures, but measures of gratitude sometimes continued long after. Beck showed me a photograph a former patient had sent him a few years after her surgery. She was posing in front of a wooded waterfall, flashing a huge smile. "You're not going to get that from a breast aug," he said with a knowing grin. For him there was a fundamental difference between a breast augmentation—and the patient who requests and undergoes it—and facial feminization surgery. A patient who gets a "breast aug" may be grateful to her surgeon, but it is not likely that her gratitude will form a long-lasting emotional link between them. The face produced through FFS enables a radical shift—predicated on a radical realization of a desired life—for which his patients' gratitude endured. For Beck the waterfall photo said a lot. It sat in his windowsill, neatly framed.

Patients' gratitude to Ousterhout sometimes verged on adoration. His global reputation for FFS made him a kind of celebrity among trans- women who visited his office, as well as many I met elsewhere. As I waited in the examination room with Darla before her initial consultation, she fidgeted and chatted nervously. She had traveled from New Zealand for her consultation with Ousterhout, and she almost bounced with anticipation. She was excited about finally making the trip she had been planning for months and finally getting the surgery she had been planning for years. More immediately she was excited to meet Ousterhout in the flesh. Darla was one of several patients who asked to pose with him in photographs, sometimes before surgery and sometimes after. Rosa, a patient who had traveled from Italy, asked me to take her picture as she posed next to the nameplate on Ousterhout's office door. He was routinely asked to autograph copies of his book that patients brought with them to conferences and consultations. When blogging about her consultation, a former patient named Kayla wrote, "Some people idolize sports heroes, I idolize Dr. O."[10] Diane wrote in an online testimony that Ousterhout was her "private god."[11]

Patients reminded me time and again that these doctors do not *have* to help them. Beck and Ousterhout had successful careers before they began working with trans- patients and, like the vast majority of their peers, could work with patients with other kinds of medical issues. The fact that these doctors were willing to apply their expertise to help trans- people despite the ethically, morally, and medically contested status of their "condition" indicated to patients that there was something special about these doctors. But surgeons do not work alone.

The historian Joanne Meyerowitz (2002) describes the early years of medical and surgical treatment for trans- people in the United States as marked by intense negotiation between patient desires and surgeons' wills. The place of the surgeon's staff also emerged as critical in the relations between patients and surgeons. Early transsexual autobiographies such as those by Canary Conn (1974) and Mario Martino (1977) describe the poor treatment patients received from hospital and physicians' staff. When seeking help from physicians in the 1960s, Conn and Martino confronted disdainful and aggressive nurses who treated them like oddities on display. Surgeons recognize that in order to create an image of themselves as caring for trans- patients in a special way, they need to have a special staff.

Each of the surgeons I met—those who perform FFS as well as those who perform GSRS—have dedicated personal assistants who perform vital functions in their practice. Many patients mention these assistants in the same breath as the surgeon when discussing their experience with surgery; they go together. With one exception all the assistants I met were women who demonstrated a fierce loyalty to the surgeons for whom they worked. One patient named Patricia pointed out the oddity of the exception. Dr. Lubbock, an FFS surgeon in the Midwest, had an assistant whom Patricia described as a "big, Guido of a guy," with an overwhelming handshake. When we were discussing her experience of meeting Lubbock at a trans- conference, she specifically mentioned how strange it was that he would choose such as person as his assistant. According to Patricia, a big guy like that just could not make her feel as safe and welcome as the other doctors' assistants had. I would argue that the seeming oddity of Lubbock's large male assistant had to do with more than his ability to make patients feel safe and welcome. Women assistants perform a powerful role as arbiters of gender in surgeons' offices. While the doctors are ultimately responsible for the production of a feminine aesthetic, their assistants do crucial gender work with patients as they interact with them "like girlfriends."

Ousterhout's personal assistant, Mira, had worked with him for more than twenty years. Mira was a striking woman with a cosmopolitan fashion sensibility. Her mode of interaction was focused on making whomever she was talking with feel good: she was a casual forearm toucher, leaning in when she talked as though every conversation was a shared secret between friends. She agreed a lot, laughed a lot, and offered a seemingly endless stream of affirmations. Each time I arrived in the office she greeted me as though my arrival was at once eagerly anticipated and a wonderful surprise. Even though I knew that everyone she spoke with was her "angel," her "darling," her "dear," when she was talking with me I felt she really meant it. Her energy and enthusiasm were astounding. She complimented shoes, she laughed at jokes, she found something to "love" about everyone and made sure they knew it.

Mira was responsible for a variety of office and patient logistics, including transporting patients to and from the hospital, helping them with travel plans, arranging translation services when necessary, overseeing Cocoon House (the private convalescent facility for patients), and managing the office's financial matters. She also performed some light routine medical procedures, such as removing sutures and changing bandages. More crucially, though, Mira performed essential emotional labor (Hochschild 1983) as she worked to create a distinct experience for patients and acted as the mediator between patients and doctor, all the while gushing over Ousterhout's abilities, skills, and successes.

The kinds of information and affirmation that Mira gave patients were fundamentally different from what Ousterhout did. Though she knew a great deal about the clinical aspects of FFS, she rarely spoke with patients about clinical details. Mira's role was to be a concerned, nonexpert woman who could convey an affirmative recognition and appreciation of femininity with patients whose own relationship to feminine bodily form had often been tenuous at best. It was Mira's job to smile, to welcome, and to reassure before surgery, and to gush, marvel, and praise afterward. As one of the first nonclinical viewers of a patient's postoperative face, Mira helped make FFS work by telling patients that it had.

When Katherine came into Ousterhout's office for her three-day postoperative appointment her eyes were bruised and blackened and she had a pale pink cast on her nose. Her thin, shoulder-length brown hair was pulled back into a loose and unwashed ponytail that bobbed along the collar of her plaid shirt. Katherine wanted FFS in order to facilitate what might eventually be a full-time transition to life as a woman. As it was, she lived her professional and family life as a man and saved her time as Katherine for weekends and the company of close friends. In the office that day she wore men's blue jeans, a roomy flannel shirt, and a pair of leather work boots. She hadn't been sleeping well. Her roommate in the Cocoon House had been either mindlessly chattering or painfully whimpering for the past three days, depriving Katherine of her rest and otherwise driving her mad.

In spite of her pain and exhaustion, though, Katherine was in good spirits. She came to the office bearing the gift of a delicate purple orchid. "Oh, this is gorgeous!" Mira exclaimed as she took the offering from Katherine's hands. "I collect orchids, you know. Every time I see this I will think of you! Thank you so much!" Mira accepted the gift and ushered Katherine into an exam room.

After her cast was removed, Katherine emerged into the main office, where Mira was waiting for her. "My god, look at you!" Mira gushed. "You are gorgeous!" A tight smile stretched across Katherine's swollen lower face. Mira continued to take her in, to admire her new look. "Do you feel amazing?" Mira asked with equal measures of curiosity and suggestion. "I'm getting there," Katherine replied, still smiling. "It's hard to tell right now, but I think it looks good." "Oh, honey, of course it does," Mira assured her. "I know it's a big change, but after a few weeks you won't even believe it."

In these kinds of interactions Mira played a vitally important role in making FFS work. She supported Ousterhout's positive narration of surgical results, but she also reflected a woman-to-woman intimacy and assurance of femininity that Ousterhout simply could not. In her interaction with Katherine, Mira looked past the very characteristics that others interpreted as signs of suspicious maleness to validate Katherine's womanhood. She looked past the men's clothing, the unwashed and unkempt hair (shampooing is forbidden in the days immediately following surgery as sutures and staples in the scalp are beginning to heal), the massively discolored bruises, swelling, and obvious fatigue, to see Katherine as "gorgeous" and to tell her so. In the early days following surgery these kinds of exchanges do more than bolster a patient's confidence; they also help patients understand their surgery was successful. While their face is still bruised and swollen and sutures are still in, while casts are on and shaved hair is still waiting to grow back, positive narrations are powerful things. Mira was one of the first people a patient saw outside the convalescent facility, and, crucially, she engaged them in exchanges about their face that were focused on their effect on her as a viewer. Though a patient could not yet know what kind of feminization the procedure had produced, Mira already did. She told patients how they looked.

Beck's assistant, Jasmine, played a similar role in his practice, but she went about her work with a much more casual affect. Her slow and easy movements were confident and elegant. She, like Mira, was a people person. When Beck prepared to give his presentation at a trans- conference,

I watched Jasmine walk into the room carrying a bouquet of flowers so large it obscured her face. After she carefully positioned the flowers on a table among pink and purple brochures and butterfly-cut sugar cookies frosted and sprinkled in purples and pinks, she turned to flash a smile at the small but eager audience. Later that evening I shared a dining table with Jasmine, Beck, and several other conference participants. We drank wine, complained about the overcooked salmon, and watched a truly entertaining *Star Trek*–themed talent show produced by the conference organizers. Jasmine moved deftly among conversations at the table. She leaned close to Beck throughout the meal to remind him of the names and personal details that helped him appear attentive and invested in each person with whom he spoke. Because the conference was a significant marketing opportunity for Beck, it was important that he make a good showing. Jasmine was essential to this effort.

Assistants like Mira and Jasmine also served as walking symbols of what surgeons could do. Surgeons who specialize in feminine aesthetics benefit from having attractive women as their assistants. At the beginning of a presentation of his work, Ousterhout introduced Mira to the audience: "This is Mira. She's been working with me for over twenty years. Can you believe it?" To which Mira replied in what seemed like a joke they'd done a thousand times, "I *do* travel with a plastic surgeon." She got some laughs. Ousterhout added, "Yeah, she's really an eighty-five-year-old guy! Doesn't she look great?" That drew the big laughs. Though this last comment was clearly meant as a joke, the fact of Mira's embodied femininity was an important part of the gender work she did in Ousterhout's practice. In the joking exchange Mira was leveraged as a living testament of Ousterhout's surgical ability, an example of the youthful femininity that he professed to produce. It helped to release the tension many anxious audience members were undoubtedly feeling, and it drew attention to femininity as a surgically producible form, playfully suggesting the very transformative capacity the audience was there to witness.

SURGERY ISN'T ABOUT MONEY IF YOU HAVE THE MONEY TO PAY FOR IT

In all of the discussions of intimacy and surgical magnanimity that surrounded Ousterhout and Beck, one topic that neither patients nor surgeons ever addressed directly was the role that money played in structuring the doctor-patient relationship. In addition to being "friends to the community," "geniuses," and "compassionate souls" these doctors were also making a very handsome living from the procedures they performed. Foregrounding FFS as an act of restitutive intimacy depended, in part, on excluding profit as a surgeon's motive. Though others sometimes accused surgeons of opportunism (more on this in chapter 4), patients I met in surgical offices asserted the beneficence of their motives.

Jill, who declared that Ousterhout "had no peers," was aware that others were sometimes critical of his work, suggesting that he had enriched himself from the suffering of trans- women, and she felt compelled to come to his defense. "Doug is a golden age," she said. "Those of us who are fortunate enough to see him will forever be a minority of people who have changed the world of opportunity for transgender people. I don't care [what others say], and I will argue that with anybody, anytime, anywhere. What he did is he opened doors that never would have otherwise been open. I never would have transitioned without coming to see him. Coming here was day one. It was a physical change, it was a mental change, it was a psychological change. It was the impossible becoming possible. He makes things possible. He is possibility." Jill's praise for Ousterhout blurred the lines between his technical work and the ethical context in which he did it: he was good not only because he was a talented surgeon but because he did his work with trans- people in a way that recognized their particular needs. She described Ousterhout's work with his trans- patients as an intimate and personal engagement that went above and beyond the expectations of a surgeon. "He has always been a friend to the community," she said. "He has given back. He has given his soul. He has given his work. He has made it his life to give other people life." Jill's account of Ousterhout's work completely elided the money he earned in the process, emphasizing instead what the effects of his work enabled for those trans- women who could afford it.

The topic of money was a very delicate one throughout my work in surgical clinics. Though I was allowed access to examination rooms and operating rooms and took part in conversations about patients and the practice more generally, the only time I was asked to excuse myself from a conversation was when finances and fees were being discussed. Ousterhout asked specifically that I not include the fee for his services in any of my writing on this project. In fact he almost never spoke of money. Neither did Beck. After performing extensive patient evaluations in which they described surgical procedures in great detail, doctors took patients to their assistants to talk about what these procedures would cost. "I give you the good news," Ousterhout would say. "Now Mira will give you the bad news."

Mira and Jasmine did give patients the bad news. They also handled deposits and payments. There are many reasons why this division of labor makes practical sense. In a private practice that depends on a steady stream of new patients, the doctor's time is better spent seeing patients than discussing finances. That said, this division of labor also allowed the doctor to keep his hands clean, as it were, to avoid the money taboo (Peltier and Giusti 2008; Stein 1983). There was a break—a literal change of location—between the place where the doctor worked and where the money changed hands. In both cases, after the doctor escorted the patient to the assistant's office, he left the room to allow the discussion of money to happen without him. This separation helped to prevent the exchange of money from turning acts of intimate care into fee-for-service commodities (May 1997).

I had expected to hear at least a few patients express frustration or resentment at the cost of FFS, which can range anywhere from $3,000 to over $60,000, depending on the procedures being performed and who is doing them. But this sentiment never came up. Not once. Instead patients took the cost of surgery as a matter of fact—good care costs money—and worked to find ways to finance it. They used their inheritance, borrowed from retirement accounts, cashed in stocks and other investments, borrowed money from friends and family, went into staggering credit card debt, took on second jobs, or simply saved up for the procedures they most desired. Once the financing was in place, they could receive the kind of high-quality, deeply intimate surgical work they longed for.

OTHER SURGEONS' POCKETBOOKS

Narrating the surgeon-patient relationship as compassionate, beneficent, and restitutive was the privilege of those who had money to pay for it. Despite the exchange of a significant amount of money, surgeons and patients discursively excluded money from the story of FFS, changing focus instead to patients' desire for transformation and surgeons' ability and willingness to enact it. While patients acknowledged—and sometimes struggled with—the cost of their operations, none of them expressed resentment toward their own doctors, though they sometimes cited the high prices of other doctors as one factor that impacted their selection of a surgeon. The only times I heard accusations of the corrupting power of money inside the surgical clinic were when surgeons criticized the work and spurious motivations of their peers. While Ousterhout and Beck were quick to assert their own beneficent aims as good surgeons, they used the contaminating specter of the profit motive to cast aspersions on others as technically proficient but ethically suspect.

The first of these instances occurred in the operating room. Ousterhout was performing a few minor revisions on Shelby, whose full-face FFS he had done several years earlier. According to Ousterhout, Shelby had been quite pleased with the results of her initial surgery.[12] Some years after that operation she had accompanied a friend to the offices of Dr. Crabtree, a leading American genital sex-reassignment surgeon who had recently begun performing FFS as well. During her friend's consultation, Crabtree remarked that Shelby could benefit from the addition of cheek implants and some revision work on her nose. Shelby agreed with his assessment and underwent the procedures he recommended. As soon as she healed from the surgery, Ousterhout told me as he pulled a translucent silicone implant away from her cheekbone, Shelby regretted having the work done. She returned to Ousterhout to have the implants removed and to have her nose (re)reconstructed into the shape Ousterhout had made during her initial FFS. Ousterhout shook his head as he dissected Shelby's nose in preparation for the rhinoplasty. He told me he could understand why Crabtree had wanted to redo Shelby's nose; noses are a matter of aesthetic taste. But "the only reason to put cheek implants in someone who doesn't need them is to line your pocketbook." In Ousterhout's estimation, Crabtree—with whom Ousterhout had a collegial and long-standing personal relationship—had taken advantage of Shelby by recommending something that, according to Ousterhout, she clearly did not need. Ousterhout described Shelby's second surgery as pure opportunism for which she would have to pay twice: once to Crabtree to put implants in, and then to Ousterhout to have them taken out.

The second occasion in which I heard one doctor accuse another of operating out of greed occurred over dinner at a conference. Beck and I shared a table with several other people at the back of a large banquet room. Despite our distance from the stage, the musical numbers being performed at the conference talent show were loud enough that we had to lean in close to each other to talk. Beck was describing what he thought made his approach to FFS different from other American surgeons. As opposed to the standardized approach he attributed to others, he described his approach as one that took patients' individual needs into account. "Not everyone needs everything," he stressed. "A doctor who does every procedure on everyone is doing it for their pocketbook and not for the patient."

These accusations call the motivation of other doctors into question by foregrounding the financial rewards that come with performing multiple procedures. Though surgeons acknowledge that practitioners have varying opinions about which procedures each patient needs in order to be sufficiently feminized, there is still an imagined standard of appropriate and inappropriate practice in this regard. In claiming that other doctors are motivated by selfishness and greed, Beck and Ousterhout identified themselves as beneficent caregivers motivated by the sincere desire to help their patients, not to be bankrolled by them. Taking personal advantage of trans-patients' desperation is bad surgery. The specter of financial gain threatens the purity of beneficence that surgeons claim motivates *them*—though it may not motivate the other guy. By locating the desire for gain elsewhere, they shore up the steadfastness of their commitment to benefit and do right by their grateful patients, not themselves. The purity of motive is a crucial part of the restitutive intimacy that saturates and animates the practice of FFS.

Historical and ethical dynamics pervaded the clinical space of trans-medicine. They shaped surgeons' experience and understanding of their work and patients' desires and expectations of the surgical interaction. They shaped how FFS was performed and how and by whom its efficacy was interpreted. In this "geography of care" FFS worked, and thus the forms of womanhood to which it laid claim were enacted, when affective and physical transformations happened together. When they did, doctors and their staff established credibility to narrate results into coherence and to make claims to efficacy that might otherwise have been left open for interpretation. It is in this sense that the affective relationship becomes a surgical technique, a way of enacting woman and helping a distinct trans-therapeutics to cohere.

Without the carefully crafted displays of intimacy so central to how prospective patients decide on surgical services, the efficacy of FFS can begin to fray at the edges. Narratives of shared motivation between patient, surgeon, and staff that made particular clinics attractive before the operation must be pulled through and presented again after the operation, now in the form of a shared reception of results. This narrative coherence makes FFS work; it pays out the promise of just motivation and makes it clear that all parties have been working toward the same end all along. Care turns the cut into an act of intimacy, becoming its accomplice in the enactment of woman.

Despite their many fans, surgeons and FFS more generally also have critics and detractors. The claim that a change in facial structure can enact a change of sex is not accepted everywhere. And even when it is accepted, it is not always considered a good thing. Sometimes FFS's claims to the performative enactment of womanhood are refused.

4 · Recognition and Refusal

After all, under what conditions do some individuals acquire a face,
a legible and visible face, and others do not? There is a language that
frames the encounter, and embedded in that language is a set of norms
concerning what will and will not constitute recognizability.
—JUDITH BUTLER, *Giving an Account of Oneself*, 2005

So far my examination of FFS has stayed close to the clinic, close to the surgeons who perform the procedure and the patients who undergo it. Inside the clinic FFS is treated as a commonsense necessity. Patients didn't need to explain why their masculine face was problematic; they needed only to present themselves to the surgeon, to turn their face up to his overhead light. The common sense of FFS goes like this: What makes a person a woman (or a man) is not the shape of her genitals but the fact that she is seen and engaged as a woman (or not) by others in her everyday life; her sex/gender is a product of ongoing social recognition and interaction, not a simple description of her reproductive anatomy. Because *woman* is a social identity reserved almost exclusively for those occupying bodies read as female, so long as others see a trans- woman's body as a male body, she cannot accomplish the goal of her transition, which is to transform her identity from man to woman. Since her face is the site of her individual identity and the part of her body that others see and engage the most in everyday life, changing her identity depends most crucially on changing her face (see Edkins 2015; Talley 2014).

What distinguishes FFS from other trans- specific surgeries is the primary role it gives to the social life of the body. Faces are meant to be seen; they are the primary bodily location of our identity as individuals and members of social groups. Operationalizing a performative account that moves sex/gender out of the properties of atomized bodies and into the realm of social intercourse means that the effects of FFS are settled in social exchanges too; it works when others see post-op patients the way surgeons and patients hope they will. Faces are assessed in the consultation room and are reconstructed in the operating room, but the question of whether FFS produced its desired effect is answered everywhere else.

Patients and surgeons located the efficacy of FFS in everyday scenes and interactions that invariably starred two players: the patient and some viewing other. The first other was the surgeon or his assistant; they looked at a patient's postoperative face and told her how she looked.[1] Later the other was someone else: a delivery man, a shop worker, a potential romantic interest, a colleague, a family member. If, in these exchanges, others saw and responded to post-op patients as women, then the surgery was understood to have worked because it produced its desired effect. These scenes and exchanges—imagined or experienced—were staged as the enactment of sex/gender, the daily practices and forms of attribution by which legible womanhood was produced and by which FFS would be understood to have produced it (or not). But woman is not only an individual category; it is also a collective category and one with political stakes. Remaining tightly focused on face-to-face interactions between two people limits the effect of FFS to the individual who underwent the procedure, making it hard to see the other things that FFS does when it does or does not work.

What are the implications of the transformative power of facial surgery beyond the patient who undergoes it? How does a model of sex/gender based on recognition articulate with the genital-centric models that continue to guide American legal policy? In this chapter I step out of the surgical clinic and back from the dyadic scenes of sex/gender attribution that surgeons and patients often referred to as "passing" in order to consider other perspectives on what FFS does and does not do. Fraught as it is for a number of other reasons, passing is not a helpful tool for thinking about the effects of FFS in contexts beyond the individual patient. Instead I suggest that recognition—a framework in all its complex entanglements with subjectivity, identity, and citizenship—provides a common form by which to attend to scalar concerns that a myopic framing of FFS as face-to-face passing cannot. Recognition is a dynamic process of exchange, not a negotiation of "true" and "false" identities. Dynamic and productive, the kinds of recognition that FFS enables and those that it does not lets us see effects of FFS that a story of pass/no pass obscures and opens fissures of disconnection between how sex/gender is regulated and understood across a number of sites. Marked inconsistencies demonstrate that conflicts over how to define sex, gender, and the logics of trans- therapeutics are not simply intellectual exercises; they have real effects on bodies, they structure access to resources, and they define the terms by which transitions take place. They also make it clear that there is no single answer to the question of whether FFS works. Better questions might be: What kinds of work does FFS do, how and for whom?

I begin my exploration of these questions by looking at refusals and rejections of FFS on political grounds. According to some critics, while FFS may enable in-person attributions of unmarked femaleness, the invisibility that FFS aimed for works against a project of trans- liberation premised on the visible presence of trans- people not as normative men and women but as distinctly trans-. These critics acknowledge the transformative capacity of FFS but challenge the political implications of effacing gender difference. Next I look at what happens when the state refuses to recognize a citizen's status as female or woman in the terms by which FFS patients assert it. Being seen as a woman on the street may constitute an interpersonal enactment that is very meaningful, but it is also one that is refused at the level of the state. Prevailing American legal and policy responses to the claim that FFS enables a change of sex is simple: no it doesn't.

NO ONE NEEDS FACIAL FEMINIZATION SURGERY

I dragged an embroidered floor pillow next to where Maya was sitting at an evening dinner party. Introduced to me by a mutual friend, Maya was curious about my research and eager to share her thoughts about FFS. A politically engaged trans- woman living in San Francisco, she knew several people who had undergone the surgery. While she acknowledged that the procedures had made significant changes in some of these people's appearance, she had no interest in having the surgery herself. "I just don't need it," she said. Maya's self-evaluation of need referred both to her personal politics and to the fact that though she had never had facial surgery, she was routinely recognized as a woman.

Maya was very out and proud about the fact of her trans- identity. She was committed to a politics of visibility and felt that those who opted to undergo FFS had not embraced the empowerment that such a politics enabled. Throughout our conversation her reflections on what trans- women "needed" telescoped back and forth between assessments of the kinds of bodily changes that might be required in order for particular trans- women to be recognized by others as female and what the personal and political ends of this kind of recognition entailed. According to Maya, trans- women did not need and should not undergo surgery to make themselves palatable to those whose definitions of women excluded them. Instead trans- women needed the self-acceptance and determination to refuse the exclusions, stigmas, and negativities that are too often directed their way. They needed to embrace their trans- identity, not go to such extreme lengths to make their gender difference invisible. Maya's rote and dismissive assurance that "people can do whatever they want" was quickly followed by the caveat "but some people think these surgeons can solve all of their problems, that they can fix everything. And they can't, you know."

Maya's attitude of defiant resistance against the requirement that trans-women's acceptance depended on how well they could reproduce the narrow confines of normative femininity was one that gained steam in the early 1990s. Pushing back against the paternalistic, punitive, and heteronormative requirements of the gender clinics that monopolized trans- medicine from the mid-1960s through the 1980s, trans- activists refused to be defined by the reductive and overdetermined ontologies that medical discourse had produced about them (Califia 1997; Stryker 2008; Valentine 2007). Sandy Stone's ([1991] 2006) foundational essay, "The Empire Strikes Back: A Posttranssexual Manifesto," articulated this resistance and called for a new transsexual politics organized by a will to remain visible as trans-. For Stone "passing" and "disappearing" were not measures of trans- success; they helped to reproduce the very conditions of vulnerable invisibility that created trans- people's alienation. Instead, Stone argued, the radical act of living visibly and legibly as a trans- person had the potential to undermine pathological narratives of trans- existence and to destabilize the structures of gender upon which they—and so many other social ills—depend. For trans- women who take up this political position, transition can and should be an open and individual process rather than one directed by a clinical schema for producing normatively gendered femininity. Living visibly as a transgressively gendered trans- person, they argue, is a way to push at the restrictive boundaries of woman so that it might include more kinds of people, even those whose bodies bear distinct signs of maleness (Bornstein 1994; Wilchins 1997). In this political milieu FFS, an intervention intended to allow trans- women to efface their visible gender difference, has been a wedge between individuals who seek to manifest their sense of self by reproducing the norms of desirable femininity and those who feel that such a project works against efforts that leverage visibility as a path toward political recognition of trans- people as a collective.

THE PLACE OF RECOGNITION

The kind of recognition FFS patients wanted was the kind that happened in everyday interactions, the little gestures and utterances by which their identity as women would be made real through citation and ratification. Following theorists of recognition like Charles Taylor (1994) and Axel Honneth (1995), we might refer to these as acts by which patients' "authentic identity" as women would be recognized. According to these theorists, the recognition of individuals' authentic identity is a good in itself and is crucial to individual flourishing and the advancement of social progress. "Misses" and "ma'ams" are therefore the forms in which an ever-expanding field of recognition enables the achievement of individual authenticity and advances a social equality premised on a commonly held value of "the good life" (McBride 2013; McQueen 2015). Public restrooms have become battlegrounds for trans- recognition precisely for this reason.

Other theorists of recognition have found fault with the assumption that definitions of the good life are held in common among all people, and they have argued that focusing on individual attainment of authentic identity or redistributive justice intended to include the excluded doesn't attend to the specific situations in which particular groups are subjected to systematic discrimination and oppression. Iris Marion Young (1990) has argued, for example, that identity-based struggles for recognition must be understood as unfolding within particular forms of systematic oppression. From this perspective it matters that trans- women are a group that has been excluded from social life, pathologized, criminalized, victimized by violence, and excluded from citizenship-based rights. Their claim to recognition *as* trans- women and as a distinct group is particular to them and is shaped by the contexts in which their particular exclusions arise. Seen in this way, when, how, and within which regulatory norms a trans- woman's identity as a woman is recognized is about more than the individual herself. There is more at stake than the attainment of her individual authenticity; recognition is also an act that shifts political discourse and opens questions about the terms by which membership in the category woman is granted, by whom, and at what cost. It was in relation to this kind of collective and justice-based recognition that critics of FFS spoke about the harm that is done when trans- women go to great lengths to make themselves palatable to those whose definition of woman would exclude them—especially when those lengths invoke the troubled history of medicalization that visibility activists militated against.

FACIAL FEMINIZATION SURGERY COSTS
TRANS- WOMEN TOO MUCH

Justine and I sat talking as we waited for the "Holistic Healthcare for TGS" workshop at a large trans- conference. As other participants filtered into the hotel conference room and found seats around mauve-draped tables, Justine was not shy in voicing her disapproval of FFS in general and Ousterhout in particular. "Dr. O.? Oh, yeah. He's great. Do you know what else he is? Rich! What does he cost now? Fifty thousand dollars?" Justine grew more animated as she spoke, scoffing and waving her hands as if the numbers were irritating gnats swarming around her head. "I knew a girl—a really beautiful girl—she went to see Dr. O., and he said she needed the works. It was ridiculous. She didn't need a thing and he said she needed *everything*. And the stupid part is, she did it." To Justine, Ousterhout and other FFS surgeons were opportunists. They preyed on trans- women's desire for social acceptance by promising a surgical fix to what she saw as the explicitly social problem of transphobia. The high price tag attached to FFS had broader ethical implications as well.

"It's so expensive," Justine went on, "that you get one little group who can afford this surgery that they say everyone just *has* to have. You watch how many girls [at the conference] will go see these surgeons talk. Well, not everyone can have FFS. Not everyone wants to have it." Justine was not alone in her criticism that expensive out-of-pocket procedures exacerbated class divides, nor in her suspicion of surgeons' motives. Another conference attendee named Karen called foul on FFS surgeons' claims to be beneficent "friends of the community." "If this surgery is so important, and they care so much," she said, "then why don't they do any pro bono operations? If this is so lifesaving, why don't they do it for all these [trans-] girls working the streets, the ones whose lives really need saving?" Karen's critique is one I heard many times. The Stanford surgeon Donald Laub, for example, traveled abroad doing pro bono cleft palate repairs in underresourced countries, but when it came to doing genital surgeries for the trans- population for which he purported to care so much, prospective patients were required to produce cash up front. The profit motive that FFS patients worked to cleanse from their relationship with their surgeon (see chapter 3) was a favored target among critics. As much as these criticisms took aims at surgeons, the dynamic they described also implicated a class of trans- women who could and did pay for very expensive procedures. According to FFS critics, they too were part of the problem.

Some claimed the high price of the transformation that FFS promises turns transition, like other forms of for-profit health care (Brock and Buchanan 1987), into a game of haves and have-nots, where decisions about whether to transition were pinned more to capital than anything else. People with the least access to body-changing technologies—those who could not afford expensive electrolysis, who could not afford physicians to prescribe and oversee their hormone use, who could not afford expensive surgeries—ended up occupying the most visibly gender-divergent bodies and thus suffering the worst stigmas and social punishments, while rich trans- women who were already in a position of relative privilege could pay to get out of such exclusions and violence.

But it wasn't just FFS to which resourced people had disproportionate access. Transition can be a very expensive process. Psychotherapists, endocrinologists, hormone prescriptions, ongoing hair removal, insurance copays, and various surgical interventions cost money and time, especially for those who don't live in or near areas where these resources are available. While it was the request for medicosurgical interventions that once constituted the diagnosis of transsexualism—thus rendering a transsexual person legible as such (Hausman 1995)—critics have argued that a treatment-based definition excludes and invalidates those people who either cannot or choose not to undergo hormonal and surgical treatments. Trans- authenticity should not be reserved exclusively for those who can afford it, they argue (Currah and Moore 2009; Gehi and Arkles 2007; Spade 2015). As the most expensive transition-related intervention, FFS was a favored target among those critical of the class and race hierarchies that allowed some resourced trans- women to cultivate an embodied form of woman that was idealized by many but available only to a few.

Justine's analysis of need in relation to FFS was committed to a trans-politics of visibility much like the one that Stone's essay imagined. It was also one that saw trans- issues as essentially linked to larger movements for social justice (Feinberg 1992). Justine knew that others did not see her as a woman, but cultivating that recognition was not her priority. More than that, she needed to do radical political work, and she understood her willingness to stand out as a transgressively gendered person as part of that work (Stryker 1994). To her no one needed FFS. And the only people who truly benefited from it were the surgeons who transformed trans- women's deep longing for personal recognition into personal wealth, all the while calling it "help."

It wasn't only critics who were aware of and conflicted about the privilege that FFS required. One of Ousterhout's patients, Jill, knew that undergoing surgery to be recognized as female—what she referred to as passing—was a contentious issue and that the ability to do so depended on having access to money that many trans- women did not. Still Jill knew that FFS had utterly transformed her life and made her dreams come true. She refused to hear criticisms of Ousterhout, of his style, of his technique, of his high price: "People can say, 'Yes, but not everyone can afford it.' I agree and that's a shame. My dad passed away and left me some money and I was fortunate enough to be able to afford what [Ousterhout] could do for me. That being said, what he did is he opened doors that never would have otherwise been open. I never would have transitioned without coming to see him. Coming here was day one." Jill's short statement demonstrates how the ethics and politics of recognition get linked to the cost of FFS. She acknowledged that FFS was out of the financial reach of many but quickly shifted the focus to the positive changes the procedure had produced in her life. Money allowed her to afford FFS, and FFS realized her identity and physically manifested her sense of herself; it allowed her to transition, to make the impossible possible. Though it may have been affected by a contested means, the arrival at her desired end—the self-actualizing materialization of her sense of self—was an end whose ethical validity, she believed, should speak for itself.

Another patient, Rachel, also grappled with the question of whether having FFS in order to "blend in" was a "moral thing to do" and how she should reconcile its morality with its high price tag:

A lot of people would say, "Oh, you're just falling into a trap. You're just furthering the gender binary. You're a dupe. You're playing into the game." That whole thing. And it certainly has some weight. You consider it. You talk about it. And the question of the gender binary. . . . I think probably most of us in the community recognize that there are more than two genders, but that doesn't necessarily mean that we have to want to be all of them. I might want to be part of what used to be called the binary, even though I recognize that there are gender-queer people who don't make that choice, who reject that choice. I totally respect that. I considered that for a while. I thought of that as a possibility. Maybe I can be sort of a new gender, a different gender. I don't have to subscribe to one or the other. But, for me, that's not really what I wanted. Theoretically it was interesting, but emotionally and psychologically it wasn't satisfying. At a certain point I just said to myself, "Really, the truth of the matter is, I just want to look as female as I possibly can. The rest of this stuff is very interesting, but that's really what I want."

Rachel knew that undergoing FFS opened her to criticisms of "playing into the game," of buying into the idea that there are only two sex/gender configurations, male/masculine and female/feminine, and that she had to choose one. She knew that many saw "furthering the gender binary" as an act of treachery and harm, but she refused responsibility for this. The possibility of upsetting gender norms—of living and presenting as genderqueer the way Justine did—was theoretically interesting, but what Rachel ultimately wanted was to "look as female as [she] possibly could."

Rachel had once felt guilty about her desires and especially her sense that fulfilling those desires would implicate a willful ignorance of the privilege she wielded. Over time, however, her sense of guilt and obligation melted away and she resolved to put her own needs first:

If I can pull together fifty thousand dollars I'm not going to feel guilty about it. There's all this thing of not everyone can afford it. Obviously. It does create a kind of divide in the community. There are certain people who can't afford it. Some of it has to do with age. I'm fifty-five years old. I accumulated a little bit of capital. I couldn't have afforded to do this when I was twenty-five. I didn't have fifty thousand dollars in the bank [then]. And there are probably plenty of twenty-five-year-olds who have a million dollars in the bank. So, it's all relative.

Rachel had taken to heart the criticisms of FFS, but she defended her choice as reflecting her personal desire for transition. Unable to reconcile her desire and decision with class- and privilege-based critiques, she ultimately decided to deny their political implications completely. "I finally said, 'This is not political. I'm not taking a political stance, here. This is about me wanting to be a whole human being. This is about me wanting to be myself. I'm not fighting for my rights. I just want to live my life.'"

Individualizing the practice of FFS was precisely the kind of move that Justine, Karen, and Maya saw as denying its political valence and thereby damaging efforts toward political progress for trans- folks.[2] Not only did the financial cost of FFS undermine community solidarity, but seeking the kind of individually affirmative recognition reserved for normatively gendered people, they argued, contributed to the stigmatization and abjection of those trans- women whose body is markedly gender-variant—often the very same people who cannot afford, do not have access to, or choose not to undergo expensive body-altering surgeries. Narratives of individual transformation and personal authenticity obscured systematic exclusions of class and race that made American FFS an intervention for resourced patients, an application of largely Caucasian standards of femininity performed on a largely Caucasian group of patients. Asserting the power of trans- visibility, FFS critics felt that when resourced trans- women opted for individual recognition of their claim to authentic womanhood, the possibility of collective and expansive political action for all trans- people was diminished.

Critics focused on what that personal desire for gendered recognition of individual authenticity meant at the level of the political. Emphasizing the transformative political potential of being recognized not as normative and respectable women but as the kind of powerfully abject and defiantly visible trans- women of Stone's essay, critics of FFS rejected the underlying premise that womanhood was dependent on recognizable femaleness. They rejected the idea that access to the category woman ought to be determined by the assessments of those operating in a gender system that consistently denied and perpetrated violence against those who did not fit its norms.[3] One should be recognized and affirmed as a woman not on the condition of occupying a normatively female body, they argued, but as the result of naming oneself a woman. Period.

Scholars of liberal political systems, especially those hoisting the banner of multiculturalism, have argued that the kind of political recognition predicated on and offering the promise of inclusion and tolerance cuts both ways (Smith 1997; Smith 2007; Sullivan 2007; Taylor 1994). The "cunning of recognition," Elizabeth Povinelli (2002) argues, is that the price of being recognized as worthy of personhood, of rights, and of citizenship is the adherence to an impossible standard. It requires that one be different enough to enrich the self-congratulatory mosaic of multicultural difference, but only in ways that reinforce existing ideas about the kinds of subjects worthy of the goods of political membership. Taking a similar tack, the philosopher Paddy McQueen (2015:144) writes of the cost of trans- inclusion, "Exclusion cannot be addressed through simple assimilation if the cost of that assimilation is a thoroughgoing erasure of the very feelings, experiences, physical attributes and beliefs which identified that individual as 'deviant' in the first place."

Demands that trans- women appear convincingly female as a condition of having their womanhood recognized is one way that such erasures take place. "Those in power not only have the ability to offer recognition to the minority group or individual," McQueen (2015:144) writes, "but also to control the terms of that recognition." Trans- women are allowed into public spaces and discourses only when and if they present themselves in ways that the dominant culture demands of those it considers legitimate. There is space for beauties like Janet Mock, Laverne Cox, and Carmen Carerra on one hand, or safely fictionalized portrayals of trans- people by nontrans-actors like Jeffrey Tambor in the series *Transparent* or Felicity Huffman in the film *TransAmerica*. But everyday trans- women who are not beautiful, are not celebrities, who do not have racial, class, or education privilege, experience forms of recognition that "undo" them: their maleness is asserted and their claims to womanhood denied (Butler 2004). The double action of refusal and denial cannot simply be understood as a failure to pass. It has to be seen as itself a productive event; it helps to create the conditions within which FFS becomes a highly desirable intervention.

FACIAL FEMINIZATION SURGERY DOESN'T DO
ANYTHING: MATERIALS OF LEGAL RECOGNITION

While some politically minded trans- women criticized FFS for what they saw as its damaging assimilationism, the individual efficacy of FFS was also challenged by American legal and policy institutions that remain committed to a genital-centric definition of sex and of surgical sex change. For this audience the face-to-face recognition of sex that doctors and patients often described as passing and to which adherents to a performative model of sex/gender attribute the power to produce embodied sex/gender as such was quite irrelevant. The state does not recognize sex based on interactions on the street; the state keeps sex in documents and enforces it through policies that significantly impact citizens' daily lives. This is especially the case for trans-folks whose body contrasts or conflicts with the documents that track them (Beauchamp 2009; Cantú 2009; Currah and Mulqueen 2011). Despite what FFS surgeons and patients say, American legal and public policy institutions do not recognize facial reconstructive surgery as a meaningful transformation of sex.

In the United States individuals are assigned a sex at birth, generally based on the appearance of their external genitalia. Sex designation is a legal artifact, marking an identifying characteristic of the body that has largely been considered permanent—except when it is not. Policies regulating whether and how sex can be changed on state-issued documents such as birth certificates and driver's licenses have varied widely over time and across jurisdictions (Beauchamp 2009; Currah and Moore 2009; Meadow 2010; van Anders et al. 2014). U.S. courts have also stipulated acceptable forms of surgery or documentation depending on whether the person requesting a change of sex designation is a trans-man or a trans-woman (Markowitz 2008; Meyerowitz 2002; Ohle 2004). As of this writing, some states require proof of surgery from the operating surgeon in order to change a citizen's sex designation on a birth certificate.[4] Others require only a letter requesting such a change. Some will not change sex designation on a birth certificate for any reason (Lambda Legal 2015). Although those states that require surgery as a condition of changing documents vary in what kinds of surgery they require and how proof of such surgery is to be presented, none accepts FFS as a surgical transformation of sex.[5] Defined and determined by an ideal of "permanent" (Currah and Moore 2009), genital-centric, and binary sex—or what van Anders and colleagues (2014) call "newborn bio/logics"—surgical requirements for changing sex designation are predominantly focused on genital surgery.[6] Based on an essential and genital-centric understanding of sex and sex change, claims to the performative efficacy and centrality of facial reconstruction that FFS advocates claim as common sense make no sense at all.[7]

In the close and controlled monitoring of bodies and identities, medical and legal authority often work together toward the aim of "correcting" trans-people's bodies into those that are coherently recognizable and countable (Spade 2003; Stryker and Currah 2015). But counting as an instance of "male" or "female" is not so simple, as requirements for legibility stretch across a range of interactions, documents, and bodily forms. A person may look quite different on the street than in official documents, and forms of recognition marshaled by the state to identify citizens may contrast sharply and dangerously with those moments of recognition exchanged between individuals based on their perceptions of bodily form (Beauchamp 2009; Cantú 2009; Currah and Mulqueen 2011). In addition to the everyday activities that require agreement between perceived sex and state-issued documentation, securing a state ID is also a means to secure rights to state-based benefits and services. "Birth certificates, for example," Currah and Moore (2009:116) write, "are not simply mechanisms for managing populations and the state enforcement of obligations, like taxation or conscription, on individuals; they also create recognition for the distribution of resources from the state to individuals, such as voting, social security, Medicaid, marriage rights, and welfare benefits." How sex and sex change are defined and how those definitions bear on models of trans- therapeutic logic can have profound effects on who gets to transition and what transition means.

What happens when parties disagree about how to define sex, and therefore how to define both the reasons for which trans- people seek medico-surgical intervention and the corresponding services offered in its name?

THE INSTITUTIONALIZATION OF A GENITAL-CENTRIC TRANS- THERAPEUTIC

Although trans- health care is undergoing rapid shifts as I write, what hasn't changed in over sixty years is that the prevailing institutionalized model of medical transition in the United States is focused on genital surgery. Long managed by individuals seeking services and the clinicians who provided them, this genital-centric model is being retrenched in health care policy even as public and private insurance coverage for trans- folks is expanding.

In May 2014 the U.S. Department of Health and Human Services (DHHS) reversed a National Coverage Determination (NCD) made in 1981 that had declared "the surgical procedures and attendant therapies for transsexualism" to be "experimental" and therefore not eligible for federally administered Medicare services.[8] The 1981 declaration had determined the way trans- health care was organized for decades. It set a lasting precedent for the exclusion of trans- medical coverage by public and private health insurance providers who argued that, as "experimental medicine," transsexual surgery was not "medically necessary" and thus not a covered benefit.[9] Experienced surgeons who were leaving university clinics for private practice in the early 1980s ended up serving patients who had the financial resources to pay surgical fees out of pocket. Less resourced folks turned to a rapidly emerging black market of illicit practitioners whose services grew in demand as institutional supports fell away (Denny 2002).

In May 2014 the DHHS reversed the 1981 policy by declaring, "Transsexual surgery *is* an effective, safe and medically necessary treatment for transsexualism" (U.S. DHHS, 2014:1, emphasis mine). This was a remarkable change in policy, not only because it lifted a long-standing ban but also for the curious fact that it did so using a diagnosis (transsexualism) and a term for its treatment (transsexual surgery) that had not been in use for decades. In 2014 the term *transsexual surgery* was no longer in use because the diagnostic entity transsexualism no longer existed. The American Psychiatric Association had replaced it with *gender identity disorder* in 1994 (*DSM-IV*), and then with *gender dysphoria* in 2013 (*DSM-5*).[10] These changes in nomenclature were not simply new labels for the same condition. Professional consensus about how to understand and provide treatment for gender nonconformity had changed significantly since the 1980s.

While transsexualism had been conceived as a genital-centric problem with a genital surgery treatment, the currently accepted diagnosis of gender dysphoria refers to the clinically relevant distress that some gender-nonconforming people experience. It does not pathologize the desire to alter bodily sex characteristics as transsexualism had done, nor does it pathologize identity as the intervening diagnosis of gender identity disorder had done. Instead gender dysphoria recognizes that living as a gender-nonconforming person can cause clinically relevant distress for some people (Zucker et al. 2013). Some people diagnosed with gender dysphoria seek genital surgeries to alleviate this distress; some do not. Some seek out hormones, chest or breast surgeries, facial surgeries, hair removal or transplant. Some seek no medical intervention at all.[11]

Though the clinicians and medical literature cited to support the 2014 overturn make note of the sweeping changes in trans- medicine since 1981 by using contemporary language, the policy document itself does not. Rather than drafting a new policy with updated language that reflected the current best-practice treatment models, the 2014 NCD simply invalidated an old one. The confirmatory statement, "Transsexual surgery is an effective, safe and medically necessary treatment for transsexualism," is not just bafflingly anachronistic; it also has implications for people seeking medical and surgical treatments appropriate to the broad and flexible understanding of contemporary gender dysphoria but whose coverage applies only to the genital surgeries that counted as transsexual surgery back in 1981.

At once new and very old, current policy delineations define genital surgery as "medically necessary" for trans- people, and other interventions as "cosmetic" in nature. Here is one example. Citing the 2014 Medicare decision, New York State revised its Medicaid policy to cover "transgender related care and services." Its coverage for "gender dysphoria treatment" includes hormones and "gender reassignment surgery." The law specifically excludes coverage for what it calls "cosmetic surgery, services, and procedures." These include but are not limited to "(a) abdominoplasty, blepharoplasty, neck tightening, or removal of redundant skin; (b) breast augmentation; (c) breast, brow, face, or forehead lifts; (d) calf, cheek, chin, nose, or pectoral implants; (e) collagen injections; (f) drugs to promote hair growth or loss; (g) electrolysis, unless required for vaginoplasty; (h) facial bone reconstruction, reduction, or sculpturing, including jaw shortening and rhinoplasty; (i) hair transplantation; (j) lip reduction; (k) liposuction; (l) thyroid chondroplasty; and (m) voice therapy, voice lessons, or voice modification surgery. For purposes of this subdivision, cosmetic surgery, services, and procedures refers to anything solely directed at improving an individual's appearance."[12] Such a classification scheme affirms that in practice gender-reassignment surgery is accomplished through genital surgery and that only genital surgery is medically necessary and thus covered as a Medicaid benefit. By contrast, FFS—like breast augmentation, electrolysis (except in preparation for vaginoplasty, which would exclude not only the rest of trans- women's bodies but also trans- men who need electrolysis in preparation for surgical procedures), hair transplant and voice modification— is not about gender; it is only about improving appearance. Because the line between necessary and cosmetic procedures is also the line between covered and uncovered procedures, there are very real economic and political stakes in designating one part of the body as gender and the rest as appearance. Americans covered by Medicare and the other public and private forms of insurance that have adopted or likely will adopt its policies in the coming months will be able to access an affordable form of surgical intervention focused on one model of sex to the exclusion of others. These policies do more than affirm a genital-centric trans- therapeutic logic; they help to reproduce it by rendering other surgical desires bureaucratically illegible, "unnecessary," and excluded from insurance benefits.

FFS surgeons and patients began advocating for the treatment efficacy of FFS long before the Medicare decision. They did this in part by leaning on the transformative capacity of FFS and also by firming up a boundary between FFS and the cosmetic procedures with which it had been disparagingly associated.

"THIS IS A FUNDAMENTAL CHANGE"

Cece had undergone a full-face operation nearly ten years before we met in Ousterhout's office on a luminous spring morning. In Cece's case this meant that during a single trip to the operating room her scalp was advanced, her hairline reshaped, her brow and forehead reduced, her nose rebuilt, her chin shortened, her jaw tapered, her upper lip shortened, and her thyroid cartilage removed. "My first operation?" she laughed. "You name it and he did it. I was in the operating room for thirteen hours. I had never been through anything like it in my entire life." For Cece FFS was totally transformative. "This surgery was the single most incredible experience of my life."

On the morning we met, Cece was not her usual glamorous self. She wore a light gray tracksuit with her short blond hair pulled back from her face. She was still recovering from a jaw revision procedure five days earlier, and her lower face was taut and swollen.[13] Cece explained that her transition began in Ousterhout's office. "In my case there was no process of being Cece and then having surgery to become a more attractive version of Cece," she said. "There was David and the life that I knew as David, and then there was this surgery that in my mind began my life as Cece. The day I left my house I left a note for my wife: 'I'm leaving. I'm going to get my face done. I'm going to give this a chance.'"

Because FFS had been the first step in her physical and then legal transition—she later had breast augmentation and genital reconstruction surgery—and because it had been such a life-changing experience, Cece made it clear that for her FFS was not cosmetic surgery. It didn't simply improve her appearance.

People look at [facial feminization] surgeries as cosmetic surgeries. It's much more about enhancing quality of life or enabling life than it is about something as simplistic as improving how you look. To say that I can now engage in life in the body in which I was originally meant to be thanks to the marvels of modern science is the same as saying thanks for the ability to fix a cleft palate or the ability to create artificial prostheses that allow you to participate in life.

To me, that's what this is about. This isn't just about, "Well, I look better." This is a fundamental change. A breast augmentation for a genetic woman who happens to want larger breasts is not the same as having a breast augmentation for a transgender woman born into a male body that then enables them to exist in a body that reflects on the outside who they are on the inside. There's a huge difference. You can look at this as physical, purely cosmetic. [But] I think if you do that, you do a disservice to the work that Dr. Ousterhout does, to the bigger picture of the doors that this opens up and where this fits into the scheme of becoming.

By saying FFS is analogous to correcting a cleft palate or creating a prosthetic limb, Cece laid claim to the therapeutic legitimacy of reconstructive surgery (Gilman 1998). Her analogy focused not on psychological properties like identity or self-esteem but on phenomenological and social being in the world. Like a prosthetic, FFS enables a different engagement with life, a kind of doing and being, a style of reaching out from and with the sexed body. For Cece this kind of bodily transformation was of a fundamentally different kind than a surgical procedure that restores the beauty and desirability of youth. To that end she framed the "genetic woman" who "happens to want larger breasts" as simply wanting more of what she has already got, a desire presumably less crucial for her self-actualization.[14] Her caricatured depiction of cosmetic surgery was intended to draw a definitive distinction: FFS was not a cosmetic improvement. It didn't just change how she looked; it changed who she was and how she was in the world. Like repairing a cleft palate, she explained, FFS enabled her to fully engage in life. Rather than a difference in degree—from smaller breasts to larger, from less to more beautiful—FFS enacts a change in kind.

In spite of—and perhaps especially because of—the therapeutic logics and technical enactments that FFS and cosmetic surgery share, patients like Cece continuously worked to create a boundary between them. At stake in this distinction was the institutional and moral legitimacy of trans- medicine and of FFS as a medically necessary response to it.[15] In contrast to policies that consider gender to be a genital property and all other bodily characteristics to be appearance, Cece claimed it was FFS that changed her life, that marked the beginning of her transition and made her transition possible. FFS was fundamental to the process of realizing her identity as a woman; it was not cosmetic surgery. (For a critique of this framing, see Talley 2014.)

American health care advocates have been working on strategies to establish the medical necessity and thus insurance eligibility of FFS and other transition-specific procedures. Activists working to extend insurance coverage for FFS have contacted me to ask my help in creating a set of metric standards that could be used to determine people for whom FFS is medically necessary. With objective standards in place, one activist named Steven explained to me over coffee, it would be easier to justify surgery and make an argument for insurance coverage. "Is there something we could measure? Like a height-to-face ratio or something that we could use? Or maybe if your jaw is this wide and your nose is this wide? Some transwomen really need it," he explained. And then he told me a story about his friend who had been shy and reclusive before her FFS. "When I saw her after surgery I didn't even recognize her at first. Yeah, she looked different. But mostly she acted different. She used to sit in the back of the room and keep her head down. Now she is in the middle of everything. She looks great, but she's also a totally different person. It really changed her life."

Steven was trying to convince me that FFS ought to be considered a medically necessary response to trans- women's diagnosed dysphoria. Or rather he was trying to convince me to help him convince American insurers of this point. While I was certainly sympathetic to his cause, I declined to collaborate in an effort to produce a measurement scheme that would help to determine whose FFS would be covered and whose would not. Any such scheme, I explained, would further reify the idea that there is a single kind of female face, or even a particular female range of features. It would make the efficacy of sex recognition into a mathematical formula and obscure the roles of context and audience in the question of why, how, and for whom FFS can work. To produce such numbers one would have to either problematically ignore or problematically reproduce distinct categories of racial and age difference like those I described in chapter 1; neither effort felt good to me.

Although Steven grudgingly understood my explanation, he remained firm that one had to work within the confines of the current system and that finding a way to cover FFS for some trans- women would be better than

covering none. His interest in establishing a formula for medically necessary FFS demonstrated just how pervasive and powerful the actuarial logic
of insurance coverage is in American medicine and how thoroughly the
political economics of health care delivery have saturated understandings
of what trans- people want and need from medicine. Zowie Davy (2011:24)
has observed that such an overtly socioeconomic motivation evacuates the
principle of diagnosis as "an authentic indicator of gender variance." Instead
it reflects the realities of American health care delivery and the struggle to
make the reality of conflicting and coexisting models of trans- therapeutics
legible to systems that have long resisted them.

The strategy of proving need affords a measure of legitimacy to trans-
medicine, but by speaking the language of the insurance industry it also
unlocks financial access to surgical treatment. As groups wielding the Standards of Care promulgated by the World Professional Association for Transgender Health work to establish such need in relation to a genital-centric
definition of sex, FFS patients are scrambling to have their definitions of
sex and treatment included too. They hope to make legible to the state and
to insurers a definition of sex as a thing enacted in social life, not defined
by genital forms, and to thereby access a form of surgical treatment that
will transform their sex by making them socially recognizable as women,
regardless of their genital anatomy.

In the clinic FFS patients and surgeons describe the transformative
capacity of surgery by telling stories of dyadic interpersonal interactions.
Imagined scenes in the grocery store, in the staff meeting, and on the street
are the stuff of FFS efficacy. It is in these moments, when another person
recognizes the FFS patient as female and genders her accordingly, that her
status as a woman is enacted and the surgery is said to work. But enactments of gender both depend upon and have impact beyond the scale of
the dyadic interaction. While an analytic of passing makes it difficult to
attend to the work of FFS on other scales, I have argued that the multivalent concept of recognition makes it possible not only to attend to such
scalar concerns—recognition of and by the individual, the collective, and
the state—but to put them into conversation. As a concept that centers
dynamic intersubjectivity, recognition is ongoing and set in conditions of
power by which both parties are constituted. Individuals, collective groups,
and state powers grant recognition to others, and it is through their dynamic engagement that each is formed and re-formed. States and collec-
tives are recognized and refused just as individuals are. But as stories about

identification documents and subsidized health care that depend upon and help to reproduce legible claims to need make clear, power is not equally distributed in recognitive relations.

FFS patients ardently desired to be seen by others and by themselves as the woman they knew themselves to be. They understood that recognition was conditioned upon their discernibly female bodies. Of course recognition as a woman could be conveyed otherwise. Advocates for trans- visibility like Maya, Justine, and Karen envisioned a world in which a trans- woman's recognition both as powerfully trans- and as rightfully woman would depend only on her assertion of her identity as such. They envisioned a recognitive justice premised on a common collective history of marginalization and exclusion that reached beyond the individual attribution of woman in a closed scene of interaction. But for Jill, Rachel, and other FFS patients, this kind of visibility, while powerful, was not the kind of trans- life they wanted to lead. They wanted, as Jay Prosser (1995:488) has described the aim of "transsexual subjects," "to arrive at where one should have always been," beyond the "uninhabitable space" of the "borderlands in between" the definable positions of man and woman. They understood this arrival depended upon a face that others saw as the face of a woman.

Political theorists have conceptualized recognition as an individual process by which authentic identity is developed and self-actualization enabled, a distinctly political process by which assertions of identity are used to ground claims to redistributive justice (in the form of rights and remunerations) and as a contextually dependent process by which justice is oriented not toward universal equality but toward redressing the particular ills experienced by marginalized groups. The kinds of recognition that trans- women receive as women can be read as all of these. The effects of FFS reverberate through all of these meanings, tying personal to political projects and stressing links between the individual, the political, and the social. Scaling back from the dyadic scenes of the surgical clinic and Saturday-morning doorstep to consider the stakes of recognition in its larger political and legal contexts helps us account for what else FFS does when it works. It helps us see that recognition—as a form of enactment—is itself an important and multivalent tool.

My Adam's Apple

On the night before my first observation in the operating room, I leaned against the desk in Ousterhout's office and watched him scroll through patient photographs on his computer. He wanted to show me photos of some facial masculinization procedures he'd been working on. Though he had never received a request for facial masculinization from a trans- man, he was interested in investigating whether there might be a market for such a thing. So far, no takers. Still he thought there were opportunities to be explored. Ousterhout had performed masculinizing facial surgeries on two nontrans- males who wanted more masculine faces, and he showed me their before-and-after photographs. The differences in one of the patients were pretty astounding. Ousterhout had given this guy a big wide jaw, a square nose, and a more deeply cut hairline. He explained that the patient was a very well-built gay man who wanted a chiseled face to match his chiseled body.

When Ousterhout told me he wanted to begin marketing these facial masculinization surgeries to trans- men, I asked him why. "Why not?" he answered. "I love to do this and I'm good at it. Do you want me to give you an Adam's apple?" He spun in his chair to look up at me.

"No, thanks," I said.

"Are you sure? I'll do it for free."

Never in my life had I thought about an Adam's apple being—or not being—in my throat. While I could see why a trans- woman might want to be rid of hers, as a trans- man I believed the absence of an Adam's apple didn't carry the same corporeal meaning as its presence did. There are lots of men without a noticeable Adam's apple, and I am one of them. But Ousterhout had offered to make me an Adam's apple. For free. The offer of a free surgery was, I suppose, intended to tip the scales. But into whose favor—his or mine—was not clear.

"No, thanks," I repeated.

"Why not? Are you chicken?" he asked with a taunting smile.

"No, I really don't need one. I never get read as trans-."

"Yes, but if someone sees you at a bar," he coaxed, "and you've got a big Adam's apple sticking out of your neck, there'll be no question if you're trans-."

This was the inverse of the explanation for why trans- women need to have their Adam's apple removed. If an Adam's apple is a strong signifier of maleness that trans- women do not want, then it must also be one that I *do* want. I wasn't sure who this observant stranger in the bar might be, but one look at that Adam's apple and they'll know I'm the man they're looking for. At that moment maleness was—or could be—located right in the middle of my throat.

"That's true," I said, conceding the power of the Adam's apple, "but I still don't want one." Anxious to move the topic away from my throat and toward throats in general, I asked him how he would go about making an Adam's apple.

"I'll take a piece of cartilage from the base of your ear," he began, tugging on his ear to show me where he meant. Without thinking, I mirrored his grab and tugged my ear. It was a satisfying tug; now I knew just what he meant. All of a sudden that hunk of hard cartilage that I'd never really noticed before had incredible potential.

"Or a piece of cartilage from your rib," he went on. He offered to make my undisputable maleness of out one of my own ribs. He could turn my Eve into Adam. I am autogenic. "I'd suture it once on either side. I think it should work." He smiled so playfully that I couldn't help but smile back.

"You don't want it to move down"—he pointed at his throat and slid his finger down toward his chest—"or end up pointing to the side." His smile grew as he described this even more absurd image. Laughing, he pointed a thumb out the side of this throat to imitate a lump of thyroid cartilage sticking out the side of his neck.

"You sure you don't want it?" he asked. I declined again.

Of course I had wanted other things: nearly twenty years of bimonthly testosterone injections and chest reconstruction surgery that included a bilateral mastectomy and nipple grafts. I had that surgery and I continue to use hormones in order to have the body that makes me recognizable as a man in the world. I worry sometimes about what might happen to me if I were to lose access to my testosterone prescription. I know what the physical effects would be, but I really can't imagine how I would deal with that new body physically or emotionally. Hormones change you. Though Ousterhout's offer of a free Adam's apple did not appeal to me, it was not an absurd offer. Nor was the proposition of performing a free surgery a simple gesture. I wonder, if by some unfortunate set of circumstances, my testosterone were gone and my body began to change, if I might regret having so blithely turned him down.

5 · The Operating Room

The self may be performative—having no being that grounds its life
other than its own doing—but those performances are materially constrained.
—CLAIRE COLEBROOK, "On Not Becoming Man," 2008

By the time most patients made the trip to the surgeon's office, they had
come to think of facial feminization surgery as enacting the change between the life they had and the life they wanted. It would, they hoped, be
the end of a deep longing for transformation that had significantly shaped
their personal, professional, and financial lives for many months or many
(many) years. For these patients the present, structured by the future goal
of surgery, had collapsed into a seemingly interminable time *before* surgery.
It was a continuation of the past experience of bodily dissatisfaction and
disaffection into the "almost," the "can't wait," the "before" to which every
day following surgery would be the "after." The operating room was the
fulcrum of this fantastic act.

During my first few trips to observe in the OR, I was overwhelmed by
the activity in the place. I managed my anxiety and self-consciousness by
fastidiously recording details in a small notebook—the motions, the smells,

the conversations. Over time, as the place became more familiar and the procedures more routine, I began to experience its extraordinary complexities. Unencumbered by the anxiety that gripped patients and the demands that occupied surgeons and nurses, I went into the OR with stories ringing in my ears. I felt compelled to hold those stories and to reconcile them with the controlled brutality of reconstructive surgery, to attend to transformations that were *enabled* in the operating room but did not *happen* there. Yes, the operating room was the setting for an extraordinary exercise of surgical capacity. Yes, it was the precise location in which patients' longed-for physical transformations took place. But it was also a place whose material dynamics pushed and pulled at conceptual frameworks of embodiment and selfhood that lay at the heart of trans- body projects. In this chapter I engage this multivalence by telling the story of the operating room as I experienced it: as a place whose tender intimacies and abrasive disconnections, visceral messiness, and conceptual overcrowding are belied by its veneer of routinized control and neat, quiet discipline.

Because there is more than one thing that happens in the operating room during an FFS operation, this chapter tells more than one story. The structure of the chapter reflects what I felt: a constant tension between the theoretical tools I had for thinking about sex, gender, and bodies, and the irreducibly material and visceral facts of radical facial surgery that were being used to shape them. I punctuate the analytic and expository prose that follows with notes from my observations of Rosalind's operation. Hers was the first operation I observed; I include it because my descriptions bear an urgency and self-conscious attention to the physical acts of surgery that fell away as I became more comfortable watching and better able to predict what was coming next. I intend the prose and the interstitial notes (in italics) as a kind of conversation, an unfolding interaction between the abstract and the concrete, the body as object and subject, and sex/gender as the stuff we are, the stuff we do, and the stuff that is done to us.

Dr. Ousterhout pointed to a chair in the hallway outside his office. He turned to me and said, "I'll walk by that spot at 7:25 a.m. If you're there, you're welcome to join me in the OR. If you're not, you're not."

Rosalind had traveled from Wales to have FFS with Ousterhout. When we met on the afternoon before her operation, she was anxious—not about the operation itself but about the postoperative recovery process. "I'm scared to death," she said. "A week before my plane ride I started praying for British Airways to go on strike. I saw a patient at the Cocoon House [Ousterhout's private recovery and convalescent facility, all gendered and natural metaphors intended] all bruised and bandaged, and I've been walking around trying to think, 'Why am I doing this?'"

> *I was tired and anxious when I joined him the next morning. What if I faint? Or vomit? What if I have to use the bathroom? What if I break some rule and can never come back? I didn't think the blood would bother me, but watching the bones in Rosalind's face get cracked and sawed apart was something else. She and I had talked about this surgery for hours. I knew what all this meant to her. We walked briskly down the hallway to the surgical wing, Ousterhout in a shirt and tie covered by his long white coat, me in my canvas jacket and shoulder bag. I saw the loafers on his feet and felt like an idiot in my running shoes—I thought they'd be best for endurance.*

Rosalind had hoped to make this trip five years before, but financial issues had delayed her plans. For her, as for all patients who shared their stories with me, arriving in this office was the culmination of a long process of self-discovery. "At twenty-five years old my hair started to fall out and I thought, 'Oh no! I haven't decided whether I want to transition!'" she explained. "I tried topical creams and things to try to keep my hair, and I became pretty obsessed with it. Then I started thinking, 'Wait, is the problem that you're going bald or that you're transgender?'"

Losing her hair forced Rosalind to confront her unresolved feelings about whether she wanted to transition. Male-pattern baldness is, as its name attests, a strong bodily signifier of maleness, whose effects are difficult to undo. Going bald brought out conflicting feelings not only about her fading youth but also about what forms of gendered embodiment might be foreclosed by her avaricious baldness. Rosalind began taking feminizing hormones in 1999 and hoped that their effects would be enough to ease the anxieties she had about her appearance. She was not ready to commit to surgical alterations at that time because, she explained, she simply could not accept the idea that she was a trans- woman. "I still thought I could cure myself of being transgendered," she said. In spite of her desire to be "cured," Rosalind began taking tentative steps toward "accentuating the feminine in [her] face." She underwent facial electrolysis that produced permanent pockmarks on her cheeks and chin, only exacerbating her self-consciousness about her appearance.[1] In 2002 she had surgery to remove her thyroid cartilage (Adam's apple) and, shortly thereafter, a rhinoplasty operation to reduce the size of her nose. "That only made my brow look bigger," she lamented. "My brow is my major concern. I need my nose to match my brow. I have a kind of Neanderthal brow now. I want to do my jaw too, but I may have to skip that for now, depending on whether I can get the money together." She laughed with resignation. "I was kind of hoping Dr. O. would say that I didn't need to do my jaw, but I know it needs to be done."

After signing in at the charge nurse's desk I followed Ousterhout into the physicians' locker room, where I was shown for the first and last time where to find the supplies I needed to enter the OR. I slid my bag and jacket into an open locker. We stripped down to our underwear and re-dressed in blue scrubs, grabbing blue paper caps from a shelf near the door to the hallway. He quickly folded the bottom rim of his cap upward before tying the white paper straps behind his head. I fumbled to do the same. As we passed through the scrub room, he handed me a surgical mask and we proceeded into the OR. I knew the smell: a familiar mix of antiseptic chemicals and freshly unwrapped devices. I had been in ORs a few times before, but never standing up. At the center of the room Rosalind was lying awake on the table, being prepped by the circulating nurse (CN). She flashed me a smile.

Rosalind knew her decision to have surgery would cause complications in her professional and personal life. She presented as a man at work and at family events and planned to continue doing so until her elderly father passed away. The thought of disappointing him with the fact of her female identity was unthinkable to her. She worked in the construction trade in a small town, and living full time as a woman was simply not an option. Worries about work and personal consequences had kept her from making many changes both to her life and to her body, but she finally decided that such concerns would no longer determine her choices. "If I have to think too much about what others think, I'll never do it. I have to do this for me," she said. "I've spent twenty-five years of my life thinking about not looking like I do now. I want that to go away. Constant thinking about that ruins the mind. After this I'll be able to think of other things, everyday things."

Rosalind told me, as did many FFS patients, that it was during puberty that she began to hate her face. As she watched her "button nose" give way to the oversized nose of a pubescent boy, she taught herself how to wash her face and brush her teeth in the dark. "My mum would go into the bathroom after me and always wonder why the blinds were closed," she said. It was easier for her to relearn these daily habits than to deal with the look of her changing face in the mirror.

I stood near the wall and tried to stay out of the way as I received my instructions once again, this time from the anesthesiologist, whose distaste for surgical masks was made evident by the way his hung loosely around his chin: Do not touch anything draped in blue cloth. If you are not sure whether you can touch something, ask first. Since this is your first time in the OR, start out in your seat with both feet on the ground. If you get queasy, put your head between your knees. Once you're sure that you can stand up without us having to pick you up, you can come and observe at the table. Don't come near the surgeon's elbows.

As much as she tried to avoid contending with the reality of her body, Rosalind knew what she looked like. In early adulthood she began occasionally going out in the evenings dressed in women's clothes, a practice she really enjoyed but one that also caused a lot of anxiety. "I look pretty good," she said, flashing me a photo of herself on her phone, "but I've been busted a lot. That's not fun, I can tell you." Though she had been aggressively confronted while "out dressed," in the daytime hours her previous procedures (facial electrolysis and nose and Adam's apple surgeries) had rendered her body suspicious to those around her, as did the fact that she wore her hair long. "People see my long hair and ask me if I'm in a band or something," she explained. "They try to figure me out, ask me if I have a girlfriend. I know I'm going to have problems when I go back to work [after FFS]."

What for years had seemed to be an irremediable disjuncture between self-identification and bodily form with two gut-wrenching alternatives—deny her identification as a woman, maintain the outward appearance of a man, and suffer the emotional distress of this willful denial; or affirm her identification as a woman, adopt the outward appearance of a woman, and suffer the social consequences of occupying an abject subject position—was now inching toward resolution. If her face were just feminine enough, she could find a path between these poles, living her days as a man and her nights as a woman. She was not under the illusion that such a thing would be easy, but she wanted it utterly. Some twenty-five years after watching her face become one that made her unrecognizable to herself, she boarded a plane to cross the Atlantic and have surgery with Ousterhout.

He went immediately to Rosalind's side. He caressed her forearm, assuring her that everything would go well and that she would look beautiful. Deeply embarrassed by my presence in this unbearably intimate moment—the time and place of a fantasy Rosalind had nurtured for decades—I couldn't find a place to fix my eyes. I wanted neither to look at her nor to look away. As Rosalind spoke to the anesthesiologist and made jokes about catheters and compression garments, I stared at her fingernails: cotton candy pink against the blue-and-white-striped blanket that covered her. Ousterhout stayed by her head until she was under anesthesia. The moment she was unconscious, the feel of the operating room changed. With the presence of a guest no longer observed—I certainly did not count as one—everyone in the OR began their tasks in haste.

Surgical feminization is not pretty. During her four-hour surgery Rosalind's skin, bones, and cartilage would be pushed, pulled, burred, sawed, cut, cracked, tucked, and sutured. It is impossible to watch this deeply invasive and physically demanding process and not understand that the stakes of recognition are high. "Being inside someone's face is an incredibly intimate thing," Ousterhout said. "I would never let someone do that much work on my face, but these patients really want it. It changes their lives." Facial feminization surgery is guided by hope for future phenomenological integration and social recognition—the creation of a body that (re)presents the self.

Ousterhout announced the plan for the day. "This is Rosalind Powell, thirty-seven years old. We're doing her forehead and nose today. She wanted to do the chin and jaw, but her credit card didn't come through. Says she'll be back for those in the fall. This should take four and a half hours. She has no allergies and is on no medication." Confirming that all parties were in agreement, he began to prepare her forehead. I took a deep breath.

The problem of materiality and the relation of the body to the variously conceived mind, brain, self, or psyche has been central for scholars of sex and
gender in general and transgender in particular. Because transsexualism—
and to some extent transgenderism later—originated as a term describing
a radical decoupling and pathological incongruence between the mind and
the body, and the latter was identified as the only possible site of therapeutic intervention (Benjamin 1966), the form and mutability of the trans-
body has remained at the center of its definition. For decades it was a desire
to modify the sexed characteristics of their body that made a trans- person
trans-. In an essentialist model, when sex is understood as an empirical fact
of biological form, these kinds of change are focused on areas in which sex
is thought to inhere. But in a performative model, when sex and gender are
collapsed and understood as effects of recognition and iteration—when
the *property* of materiality is replaced by the *process* of materialization—the
place of bodily forms is unsettled, and contending with their surgical alter-
ation can be mired in multiple layers of meaning and contestation.

> *Sitting on his stool at the end of the table, Ousterhout began to comb and
> gather Rosalind's long hair in rubber bands. Once the incision site was iso-
> lated, he shaved an inch-wide track through her hair, combed out the loose
> pieces and dropped them into a biohazard bucket. He injected the incision
> site with local anesthetic and then left the room to scrub in. While he was
> out, the CN sterilized the incision site by scrubbing it with soap and water
> and then with Betadine that dripped its deep brown-yellow color through
> Rosalind's hair and into towels piled on the floor. Ousterhout returned
> with his clean and dripping hands held at chest level. The CN helped him
> into his gown and gloves.*

Because theories of performative gendering are modeled on language,
they have been named as contributing to a "turn to discourse" at the end
of the twentieth century. Scholars of gender have read this turn as both
a positive and a negative one for trans- folks. On the one hand, the de-
stabilization of both gender and sex opened the possibility for thinking of
and living these things differently. Better than that, gender transgression
became—and to some extent remains—a principal mode, and the transgender figure a principal metaphor, through which the conservative forms
of embodiment, sociality, and subjectivity can be challenged (Prosser 1995,

1998). It is no coincidence that transgender theory began to emerge alongside and in concert with this work. But there are two "on the other hands" here. First, not everyone who wants to loosen up the rigidity of the binary and naturalized gender system wants to do so or is able to do so by embodying transgression. Second, conceiving of sex/gender as performative and the collapse of the line between physical and social as one of its discursive effects meant that a new relationship between doing a gender and being a body was required. Particularly for transsexual people, whose very legibility, not to mention the medicosurgical treatments that follow from it, was constituted by a troubled relation between Cartesian body and mind, the notion that "sex is a fiction" (Butler 1993:6) was profoundly troubling. To some the very theoretical move that might have made gender and sex transgression not only possible but politically productive also seemed to undermine the transsexual claim: I am a fully constituted subject, misembodied.

Ousterhout draped sterile blue towels over Rosalind's hair and secured them in place with skin staples. Fully draped from head to toe, only Rosalind's face was showing.[2] He placed a stitch in each of her eyelids to keep her eyes closed (and thus moist) while her face was tugged and moved throughout the operation. All was ready to proceed. Ousterhout announced the time of the first incision, the CN recorded it on the whiteboard on the wall, and the operation began. Incisions started above each ear and met at the center of Rosalind's head, just behind her hairline. Her forehead skin—from hairline to orbits (eye sockets)—was folded down over her eyes like a blindfold. The raw underside of her downturned skin was spotted with the blooming red of severed blood vessels. What she called her "Neanderthal brow" was revealed now not as an effect of bone but as bone itself. So much smooth, white bone.

One of the primary criticisms of Butler's performative theory of sex/gender as a doing rather than a being is that it did not take the material body into proper account. Noting that "Butler has been charged with failing at times to make the body enough of a drag on signification," Biddy Martin (1994:110) acknowledged the value of thinking about gender as the effect of discursive performances, so long as the material body is "conceived as a drag or a limit as well as a potential" (119). In conversation with scholars working under the rubric of "new materialism," Alexander Edmonds (2013) has more recently reiterated the need to think about the ways that biologies limit and constrain agency. This is especially the case when the very sites in which essential differences in sex, gender, and beauty are biologized become targets for intervention and resignification. Specifying these sorts of "drags" and "limits" is precisely what is foregrounded in an analysis of enactment; it puts ethnographic specificity into the theory of the performativity of sex and gender, a move that tests the robustness of the theory and allows a view on the kind of work the theory does. Contending with bodily materiality has been a significant concern in the growing field of transgender studies.[3]

> Ousterhout dipped the wooden handle of a cotton swab in methylene blue dye to mark the periosteum (a membrane that lines the outer surface of bones). He cut it at these lines and scraped it forward into Rosalind's eye sockets. The bone surface was prepared. Glancing at the cephalograms illuminated on the wall-mounted light board, he used a yellow wooden pencil to mark the places where he would begin to burr and saw her forehead bone. The burr tool whirred like a dental drill as it ground down the undesirable bony prominences above Rosalind's eyes. Bone particles flew off the burr and caught in the folds of my scrubs as I leaned in. By the end of the procedure they would become dry chalky dust. Ousterhout replaced the burr attachment with an oscillating saw blade and began to cut along the pencil-drawn lines. He wedged the blunt end of forceps into the cut and pried the bone up out of its place. There was a dull cracking sound when the frontal bone was dislodged from the skull. The surgical nurse (SN) collected the irregular oblong piece of bone (about two inches across at its widest point) and set it in the white plastic lid of a sample cup for safekeeping. The frontal sinus was revealed. Frontal sinuses (95 percent of us have them) are structured differently. Rosalind's was internally asymmetrical, divided by thin walls of bone into three distinct cavities. These sinuses are usually empty, but sometimes brain matter can protrude into them. Rosalind's had filled with blood, making it hard to see what was inside. "Is that brain or sinus?" he asked no one in particular. "Not sure. Let's go slow."

One interpretation of the performative intervention conflated linguistic performativity with theatrical performance. Though Butler herself has argued that this interpretation is a misreading, this kind of theorization gained a great deal of traction in the years immediately following the publication of *Gender Trouble* (1990), drawing a focus on the body's surfaces. Theorized as performance, gender was imagined as a volitional project, something that a knowing subject could actively choose to do and undo. Like fashion, gender was play; it could be put on and taken off, artfully constructed by a willing (and well ornamented) subject (Garber 1991; see Coogan 2006). Seen in this way transsexualism was characterized as a self-fashioning project in which the self was literalized to the body. Through the election and acquisition of hormonal and surgical interventions, the body itself could be redesigned and rewritten, shed and changed (see especially Bornstein 1994).[4]

Many trans-writers have found fault with both the gender-as-performative and gender-as-performance positions, largely on the grounds that they inadequately theorize the specificity of the material body.[5] These critics claim that reading the body either as radically contingent (as in theories of performativity) or as a neutral object whose gender can be willfully donned and discarded (as in theories of performance) elides the specificity of the transsexual experience. Beginning in the late 1990s several trans- writers sought to reassert the primacy of the body on these grounds and argue that trans- subjectivity could not be understood without it (Califia 1997; Cameron 1996; Cromwell 1999; Feinberg 1998; Green 1999; Kotula 2002; Rubin 2003). In various ways these authors expressed frustration with what they saw as the obfuscating abstractions of the very theories that were celebrating gender transgression. There seemed to be much more space for the transgender figure as a site of potential and icon of transgression, but not much for actual trans- people living in time and space.

Fortunately for all there was no brain matter in Rosalind's frontal sinus. After the blood was suctioned away, the internal sinus walls were removed. Ousterhout used the burr to smooth the bone at the site of the cut and to ensure the symmetry of the previously burred sites above the orbits. He looked away as he felt for symmetry with his fingertips—burring and feeling, burring and feeling, until he was satisfied with the smoothness and symmetricality of the bone. The skin of Rosalind's forehead was pulled up to its original position, instantly turning the site from skull to face. Ousterhout looked at her face, rubbing roughly through the skin to feel for ridges in the bone beneath. He tipped her head from side to side to look at it from different angles. Tip, feel, tip, look. "Looks different to me."

He folded Rosalind's skin forward again and used saline to rinse blood and bone particles away from its raw underside. He retrieved the large piece of bone that he had removed and fashioned it into a pair of patches to cover the sinuses that its removal exposed. Each piece was held over its corresponding cavity. Excess material around the edges was marked with a pencil and burred away. He repeated the trimming process until the patch fit the cavity exactly. Exactly. Ousterhout jokingly told me, "You have to patch the hole completely because all of the sinuses in your skull are connected. If the bone is not properly patched, each time you blow your nose you'd make a bubble [under the skin of the forehead]. Each time you sniff, you'd make a dimple. That's fun at the first cocktail party, but not the second."

In my reading the richest early pushback against the abstraction of trans-embodiment in gender theory was Jay Prosser's *Second Skins* (1998). Prosser examines transsexual autobiographies with the explicit aim of reconstituting the "material figure of transition" and naming the substance of the transgender subject as "unequivocally material" (6). His opening chapter, "Judith Butler: Queer Feminism, Transgender, and the Transubstantiation of Sex," stages the text explicitly in contrast to what he reads as Butler's unmooring of the body through the assertion of the radical constructedness of sex. Prosser formulates a trans- subjectivity that is centrally configured around the contested relationship to its material, corporeal condition. His analysis acknowledges the historical origins and political effects of "wrong body" discourse but also asks that we take that discourse seriously. "The image of wrong embodiment describes most effectively the experience of pre-transition (dis)embodiment: the feeling of a sexed body dysphoria profoundly and subjectively experienced," he writes (69). Analyzing trans- autobiographies, Prosser argues that being a trans- person *is* a feeling of profound alienation or dissociation.[6] Since it is a problem of the body, it can be abated only by an intervention in the body.[7] And that body is one that matters.

Ousterhout used a yellow pencil to mark the sites where corresponding holes would be drilled in the frontal bone and in the bone patches. He threaded stainless steel nonmagnetic wires through the holes and spun them down tight. He trimmed the ends of the wires and turned them inward. The bone work on the forehead was done. Rosalind's forehead had been set back 5 millimeters. He pulled up the periosteum and sutured it together. A small, hexagonal piece of scalp was excised in the center of her head at the site of the principal incision. By removing this tissue, when the forehead and scalp are sutured together Rosalind's forehead and eyebrows would appear raised and tightened. In order to advance her hairline—and

mitigate the hair loss that so bothered her—her scalp would be moved for-
ward on her head. "This," Ousterhout explained, "is just like the Indians
did it." Tugging on the scalp he used a scalpel to cut the connective tissue
that binds scalp to skull. They came apart with an ease that surprised
me. With her forehead skin still folded forward and her scalp loosely dis-
connected from the bone, a considerable amount of Rosalind's skull was
visible. The tissue of skin and scalp were at once substantial and formless;
they looked fake, like a latex Halloween mask wrapped around hard bone.
Ousterhout pushed her scalp forward toward her face and secured it in
its new position by pulling a suture through a shallow hole he had drilled
into her frontal bone. Rosalind's recessed hairline had been remedied—at
least for the time being. Despite her use of hormones and topical creams,
her balding might continue, rendering this surgical fix a temporary one.

Notwithstanding criticisms that Prosser's and others' responses misread
Butler's project (Butler 1993, 2004; Salamon 2010), the desire to recuperate
a distinctly trans- body from the preponderance of late twentieth-century
gender theory persists. While many of the FFS patients I talked with were
perfectly able to reproduce the claim that sex/gender was a kind of doing,
they were also painfully aware that their body didn't let them do it right. At
least not in the way they wanted, in ways that others could recognize. Mostly
they experienced their body as limiting and constraining their ability to do
"woman." Such an understanding does not require an essentialist theory of
the body—FFS is about more than relocating the essentialist project from
genitals to face—nor does it require universalist claims to sexed difference.
It does have to do with the body in time and place, a body that is seen and
rendered into significance by forms of recognition in its social world. I think
this is the kind of irreducibly social and intersubjective body that trans- critics of gender theory have called for. But such calls have been resisted.

Gayle Salamon (2010:91) has recently read the "real body" of these
trans- theorists as one in which "'real' is equated with what is actual, what is
materially given, that which resists theorizing and whose existence for the
subject is beyond question." In Salamon's reading this sort of "real body" is
problematic because it is one in which the stuff of the body is posited as preexisting meaning, as though bodies—or anything else—exist in the world
first, and then language and interpretation make sense of these bodies only
as a second order of thinking.[8] Like phenomenological and psychoanalytic
theories of subject formation, performative theories of gender argue that

bodies—like anything else—come into being in and through the discursive practices that give them meaning. This does not mean the world is an empty void until I think things into being (poof!); it means that objects become recognized, defined, and important in relation to what I and others think about them; they move from being into meaning. While this argument jibes rather well in relation to gender—taken as a set of expectations about masculine and feminine behavior, affects, and affinities that change across time and place—it is less easy to make in relation to sex, taken as a set of physical properties about a flesh-and-bone organism that shares common properties with other flesh-and-bone organisms. While I may be able to change the style of my gait—and the gender and class signifiers that amble along within it—I cannot change the hips with which I walk. In the daily practice of living, those bony structures stubbornly resist my agentic efforts. I can rethink what my hip bones mean to me as signifiers of bodily sex—I can transform their meaning through affect and intention—but getting other people to share my new understanding of my physical form and to respond to me in accordance with that new understanding is something else entirely. A language known only to an individual is not a language at all (Wittgenstein [1953] 2010: §243). The body *means* socially, intersubjectively, between persons.

> Ousterhout sutured the dermis [deep layer of the skin]. The epidermis [surface layer of the skin] is sutured closed where there is no hair, and stapled closed where there is. Stapling ensures that no hair will be lost at the incision site. He coarsely combed through Rosalind's hair and began to rinse out the blood and bone particles with bottles of saline. For a moment the acrid smell of cauterized blood vessels was replaced by the sweet, tropical fruity scent of Rosalind's hair conditioner. The CN finished rinsing and then squatted down to look at Rosalind's profile. "The forehead looks great," she said. "Good job. She looks really nice." Ousterhout injected local anesthetic into the next sites—Rosalind's nose and upper lip—and left the room for a thirty-minute lunch break.

As an alternative to the body that trans- theorists desire—one that she glosses as a "nonsocial material thing"—Salamon (2010:92) offers the "real" body of phenomenological speculation. This is a body stripped of the "natural attitude" that assumes a connection between *I* and *we*, whose "realness" is constituted "by a horizon of possibility, an openness to all the different experiences that it represents to any given person" (91).

This is the second distinction between the real body thought as a nonsocial material thing and the real body that phenomenology offers; the former is real to the extent that it confirms what we already know (about materiality, about gender, about itself) and the latter is real to the extent that it points toward its own capacity to exceed what we suppose about it. To be real, in this sense, is to hold one's body and one's self open to the possibilities of what one cannot know or anticipate in advance. It is to be situated at materiality's threshold of possibility rather than caught within a materiality that is at its core constricted, constrictive, and determining. (92)

The contrast between these two kinds of "real bodies" is Salamon's own design. She sees phenomenology as in some ways attempting the kind of real body she thinks trans- theorists are calling for—one made sensible by a departure from the ostensibly shared views of the world, but doing so toward a potentially more liberating end. In making this contrast Salamon (2010:92) laments that trans- people haven't seen phenomenology as a resource for rethinking signification but suspects that her own turn to phenomenology has "responded to that call [for attention to the real body] by offering only more linguistic abstraction and speculation."

Indeed while noting that her turn to phenomenological figures like Husserl and Merleau-Ponty may be "precisely the dismissal of the real world against which critics of theoretical and philosophical approaches to gender warn us," Salamon (2010:91–92) argues that such a view "misses the purpose toward which such speculative endeavors aim." The phenomenological project is not an attempt to do away with the real world," she goes on, "but rather to question our suppositions about that world so that we might see it more clearly and utterly" (92). Salamon is quite right on this final point. Still I would argue that rarely can the world—or a body—be seen more clearly and utterly than when that body is hit by a bottle thrown from a passing car. Or pushed up against a wall. Or violently murdered. Or looked up and down before being denied vital medical care. It is not that thinking through the material conditions of embodiment is somehow *better* than thinking through the philosophical frameworks of its possibility. Rather, beginning from the lived material body as one that is located in ethnographic time and space and thinking through the implications of its social life is what calls to recenter the trans- body are about. I think there is an urgent and middle way between theorizing the body—and thus the trans- project—as radical contingency or "nonsocial materiality." That middle way is a body performatively materialized into a definite time and place. It is a historicized body enacted, one that bears the traces of the powerful discursive conditions through which it has acquired meaning but one that exists and must live within those conditions. This body is irreducibly social, irreducibly material.

> To begin Rosalind's rhinoplasty—the longest procedure in a full-face operation—Ousterhout packed her nose with cotton strips soaked in liquid cocaine the bright green color of mouthwash. He trimmed her nose hairs with small scissors. A sponge called a "throat pack" was placed to keep blood from running down her throat and into her stomach. Rosalind's nose was off the midline and had a fairly rare double septum. Interested in this feature, the anesthesiologist got up from his chair to look at the cephalogram. He referred to Rosalind as "he." The SN offered a corrective "she" under his breath. There appeared to be no notice made of the correction. An incision was made across Rosalind's nasal septum to begin the dissection of her nose. I remembered the fond nostalgia with which she had spoken of the button nose she had before puberty produced the nose that was currently being unmade. Once the front tip was dissected and pushed back (reminiscent of a pig snout), instruments were inserted under her skin all the way up to her nose bridge. I felt a pang of hope for her button nose, as my own stomach fluttered. "Now that we're done with the dissection, we need to decide what to do." Because he'd removed her frontal sinus, Ousterhout had to reduce her nose bridge. Otherwise she "would be left looking like Dick Tracy," with a sharp, bony shelf at the top of her nose, just above her eyes. He inserted an osteotome (chisel instrument) beneath the dissected skin of Rosalind's nose and slid it upward in order to reach this place. Ousterhout held the osteotome in place. Each time he said "Mm-hmm" the SN tapped the end with a small hammer. Ousterhout moved the instrument to see if the bone they'd been tapping had dislodged. He bore down on the handle of a long rasp as he pushed and pulled it across the site of the bone break. Rosalind's head nodded, as if in agreement.

Though the body in FFS is not exclusively material, it is crucially material. It was Rosalind's body—her bones and skin and muscle and hair—that got her "busted," that marked a limit to how others were willing to recognize her. Rosalind wasn't on the table because she was constitutionally unable to think her body was "situated at materiality's threshold of possibility." She may have been perfectly able to think of her body that way in the quiet moments when she leaned into the mirror and rubbed her smoky eye shadow into a damp washcloth. She was on the operating table because she had not recognized her reflection in the mirror for more than thirty years. And though others could have recognized her as a woman in some other time and place or in some other imaginable world, where she lived here and now, they wouldn't. They busted her instead. Rosalind's body problem was the one made meaningful in and through being: a material thing, irreducibly social, a product of its historical moment, and an object of technological desire that outpaced her supply of corporately extended credit. It could have been otherwise, and we could argue that it *should be* otherwise, but for her it wasn't. If how we think the body is constituted and how we understand its material properties matter as sites and forms of meaningful difference, and if the body marks a physical limit to the play of gendered signification, then identifying the conditions of that limit is a distinctly anthropological problem, one that begins with patients and their surgeons acting in the world. It demands attending to that world, in all its bloody mess.

> *Ousterhout felt through the skin between Rosalind's eyes for smoothness of the bone beneath. Blue and purple bruises were already beginning to form there. He used bone rongeurs (a tool that combines the cutting ability of scissors with the gripping ability of pliers) to remove the broken bone and cartilage. The excised pieces of cartilage were set aside in case he would need them to restructure the tip of Rosalind's nose. I was alarmed by the amount of material that was removed. He kept pulling out more and more bone and cartilage. The once-hard bridge of her nose was now pliant and moldable. He stabilized the inside of her nose with two plastic pieces, the size and shape of large kidney beans. They would remain sutured in place until her nose was "unpacked" at her five-day postoperative exam. Ousterhout opened Rosalind's mouth and tilted back her head. He made an incision where her top lip met her gum line, on either side of the center of her mouth. He inserted a long osteotome through the incision and slid it up under the skin to access the bone and cartilage that would be broken and removed in order to reduce the width of her nose bridge. "Mm-hmm." Tap-TAP. "Mm-hmm." Tap-TAP. Until all of the desired material was broken and removed.*

The stakes are high for those whose lives depend not on thinking about trans- bodies but surviving in them. Some patients wished they could be recognized as women without surgery, that a change in social expectations might allow them to move through the world looking like they did and be unimpeded by their non-gender-normative body. But this was not the world they lived in. Trans- people—especially trans- women and most especially trans- women of color—are frequent victims of discrimination and violence, the worst of which is often reserved for those people who are visibly gender-transgressive: those who *look* trans-. Sanguine calls to increase tolerance and acceptance for trans- people offer little solace in the face of these realities.

THIS BODY IS A DRAG

The ongoing practice of FFS forces an engagement with the body as a drag on the signification of gender and a limit on the ways gendered identities may be practically enacted. As the surgical discourse of FFS acknowledges, bodies are not neutral structures upon which sexually differentiated parts are draped. We don't all look the same under our haircuts, cosmetics, and T-shirts. We don't all have the same body shape with which we walk, gesture, dance, and talk ourselves into gendered distinction. Overwhelmingly the patients who sought FFS did so because these other mechanisms for enacting gender through doing—haircuts, cosmetics, T-shirts, walking, gesturing, dancing, talking—did not do for them what they'd hoped. These efforts failed at eliciting "woman" because the bodies of these trans- women were too masculine to make this performance legible to those around them. In linguistic terms, the performative was not felicitous because it wasn't recognized by the forms of authority to which it appealed; people wouldn't see "woman" where they also saw "male." And it wasn't just that these trans-women were not recognized as women; they were recognized as men trying and failing at femininity. The play of gender can and is shut down with tremendous speed and force. Embodied forms of femininity are the disproportionate target of such policing and punishment (Serano 2007).

The skin of Rosalind's nose was pulled down to assess its appearance. Seeing that more cartilage support was needed to avoid a step-down appearance from the bridge of the nose, Ousterhout used a scalpel to sort through the pile of excised cartilage and found a piece that would do. He cut it into the proper shape and thickness and provisionally placed it inside Rosalind's nose. He pressed and pinched to achieve the shape he desired. With a hand under her chin, he turned her face from side to side. "I think I got it." He placed the blunt end of a scalpel between Rosalind's two front teeth in order to establish the midline of her face and assure that her new nose was centered properly.

When we foreground the materiality of the body—and the bony skull is particularly well suited to this task—the performative claim that sex is a product of discourse rather than a given property of atomistic bodies is both useful for analysis and a solid dead end. It is useful in understanding the process by which claims to bodily dimorphism are naturalized, like the development of "the female skull" that I outlined in the introduction (see also Gere 1999). We can use this approach to see how gendered expectations have animated claims in the name of biological, evolutionary, and other sciences of classification. "Female faces" are not discrete things; they are made to seem so through extraordinary choreographies of knowledge and power. But on a daily basis, knowing that "the female face" is a historical artifact deeply entangled in histories of race, gendered aesthetics, and a dubious conjunction of scientific methods doesn't do much for trans- women who are harassed as they walk down the street. Could the story of bodily sex difference be read otherwise? Absolutely. And ethnographies of how gender and trans- identities are done elsewhere give us these productive contrasts (e.g., Kulick 1998; Ochoa 2014; Poompruek et al. 2014; Sinnott 2004). But the FFS patients I met could not make use of this transformative potential; they lived their body in a time and place that they read as foreclosing possibility, not bursting with its promise. For them the preponderance of perceived maleness in their body meant that there was no kind of doing that would make their womanhood recognizable to others. It was through historically particular forms of recognition that their claim to womanhood was foreclosed to them, and it was in relation to these same forms that they could act to claim it. Because it was surgically possible, and because it was financially accessible to them, FFS patients wanted the kind of womanhood that could be enacted in their time and place. To the extent that we understand "woman" and "man" to be social and not anatomical identities, differences between bodies make men and women possible, and social recognition is what makes them real.

Rosalind believed the activities that took place in the operating room while her consciousness was anesthetized away—the activities that you've been reading along with this text—would change her life in ways that nothing else could. "This surgery will project the internal view of me outwardly," she explained. Theorists of (trans)gender whose concerns include considering the conditions in which trans- lives may move from being "unlivable" to "livable" (Butler 2004) must be attentive to such a belief and what it motivates. This attentiveness does not mean turning away from the critical insights of queer theory or the performative theory of gendering and thinking about the body as either pre- or nonsocial. It means thinking the body *with* these insights and looking, as Austin's (1962) formulation of performativity did so explicitly, at the forms of authority within which an utterance derives its power to bring something into the world; in other words, looking at the conditions of power that make claims to embodied gender possible in a contemporary age characterized at once by a valorization of gender fluidity and an utter commitment to the rational powers of biomedicine. Both experiences of gendered embodiment and medico-scientific claims to sex difference are historically and geographically particular. They depend on existing regimes of authority that are often intensely problematic—in their reproduction of racial and class-based hierarchies and celebration of particular forms of beauty as the very definition of femaleness—and they also undeniably structure the world in which Rosalind's life, and all of our lives, unfold.

> *The nursing staff counted the sponges before Ousterhout placed the final sutures. He stood up and raised the table. He wiped the blood from Rosalind's face with gauze pads and packed her nose with wet gauze. The CN notified the recovery nurse that the patient would arrive soon. Ousterhout applied a sweet and pungent pine resin adhesive to the skin of Rosalind's nose, followed by a layer of tape. He bent the hard pink casting material over the barrel of a syringe to achieve the shape of her nose bridge. Ointment and tape covered the scalp incision, and a layer of gauze covered them. A dry gauze wrap was wound around the crown of her head. Ousterhout shook his head when he saw the pockmarks on her cheeks and chin. "No one tells them that facial electrolysis will leave pockmarks. No way to get rid of those." He removed the sutures from Rosalind's eyelids as she began to stir.*

COMING OUT OF IT

There is no way to observe in the operating room and not contend with the visceral materiality of the bodies in action there. Surgeons cut, saw, press, and grind away at bones, using all of their stamina and sensory powers to enact a well-controlled violence (Prentice 2012). Patients actively submit themselves and are anesthetically absented so that their body can be treated by the surgeon the way the patients themselves have long experienced it: as a stubbornly material and ultimately disloyal thing.

For these two people in this place, the patient's face is a plastic thing. It is not the corporeal site of personhood or individual identity; it is a series of structures whose problematic characteristics can be rectified. These structures do not necessarily map onto or even remotely relate to the social or personal identity that the face is typically taken to be. That is just the point: *this face is not her face*. Not yet at least. Rosalind and Ousterhout agreed that her face was in there somewhere, waiting to be revealed under the excess of so much bone. He took her to the OR and set about cutting it out. Apart from the debates of the ethics and politics of FFS, the forms of authority and power to which efforts for recognition appeal, the question of who can have this procedure and how it is positioned in relation to a genital-centric definition of sex and thus of trans- therapeutics, FFS is a physically transformative event.

In contrast to the undeniably corporeal and material form of woman that was materialized in the operating room, the theoretical tools I had for thinking about sex and gender had been overwhelmingly abstract: rhetorical, discursive, psychoanalytic, critical of power relations but hardly redemptive of them. They were slippery, not like bloodied cartilage is slippery but like philosophical concepts can be. In my time in the OR I felt pressed between these things—bodies and concepts—as they each made their own demands. How could I talk about FFS? How could I put such a project of sexed and gendered self-making in time and place, flesh and blood without adhering to a troubled conception of gender on one hand, or implying that FFS patients were operating under some kind of false consciousness, on the other? How could I voice the limit that FFS names when it both invokes and simultaneously refuses performative models? My humble answer to all these questions is *ethnographically*. I have tried to show you all of this at once, enactments of contradiction proceeding in time and space. Sometimes the object of ethnography is uncertainty itself, and I can get at its edges by letting the worlds of action and thought speak together not as complementary but as co-constitutive (Stevenson 2014).

The anesthesiologist leaned over and spoke loudly in Rosalind's ear: "You did a great job. Surgery is over. Just relax. Let us move you." Rosalind tried to raise her head. Her hands left the table as she hum-mumbled the amnesiac talk of anesthesia. I followed the OR nurses as they rolled her gurney into the recovery area and explained her chart to the nurses there. After Ousterhout went to check on a few other patients in recovery, I wound my way through the halls, where some passerby reprimanded me for removing my paper cap before I finally found the locker room. Once inside, I slumped on a wooden bench, exhausted and overcome.

Rosalind's body was not a stage on which to conduct an academic debate. Now stripped of my scrubs and dressed in my street clothes, I did not want to sit at some café, still smelling of antiseptic, and type out an argument for some particular political or philosophical future where trans- bodies like hers could or should be done differently. I wanted to do something more modest and, I think, more urgent. I wanted to be soberly present as trans-bodies like Rosalind's were being done, as the motions of saw and scalpel materialized her desire for "woman," enacted it right there in the room. I was in the OR differently than she was, and differently than the surgeons and nurses were (Hirschauer 1991; Young 1997). I understood what was at stake for her because I'd known what was at stake for me when I had been the patient on the table. I tried to be the kind of witness that I would have wanted for myself.

By paying ethnographic attention to actions, going into the doctor's office and operating room and being with patients and surgeons in the space of interface, I wanted to understand how trans- therapeutics—how the logic of *sex* and *gender* and the medicine meant to intervene in them—were being done in real time. It was a different project fundamentally from one about imagining, or suggesting, or hoping or willing into existence some other kind of trans- narrative. Projects of political and philosophical imagination are vital to our collective spirit; they give us something to look forward to, a future worth working for. They help us envision possibilities that have not yet existed. But the present isn't only a moment to be surpassed. Being present with Rosalind and other FFS patients meant remaining in complexity and contradiction without looking for relief and letting the gravity of this radical surgery have its way.

My time in the operating room had a profound effect on me and my understanding of FFS. The guarded skepticism I had harbored toward Ousterhout softened considerably on that first day. The man was incredibly skilled at his job. I've always been taken with skilled craftsmanship (as I peck away at my computer keyboard and dream of a life of carpentry). He took great pride in doing what he thought was right for his patients, and he did it well. Though none of us could predict the outcome of the surgery, there was no doubt that Rosalind looked significantly different when she left that room from when she entered it. Ousterhout had delivered his promise: to instantiate in Rosalind's forehead and nose his dimensions of the better-than-normal female. If she could get the funds together, he would do the same to her jaw and chin in the fall. This was, for him and for her, a crucial means for making "woman" possible.

But sex/gender is not a thing that can be said to be done once and for all.

6 · And After

The discursive condition of social recognition *precedes* and *conditions*
the formation of the subject: recognition is not conferred on a subject, but
forms the subject. —JUDITH BUTLER, *Bodies That Matter*, 1993

When a patient first encounters her new face after surgery, it is covered
with bandages, dressings, and tape. Much of the skin that is visible is taut,
swollen, and discolored. Her nose may be packed full of gauze and in a cast
from bridge to tip. There may be drains pulling blood from either side of
her newly contoured jaw. She may need to suction saliva from her mouth
because the throat pack placed during surgery will make it uncomfortable
to swallow, though she must also be careful not to induce so much suction
that the gauze from her nose is pulled down through her nasal passages and
into her mouth. For the first several days following surgery she may need to
manually stretch the muscles of her jaw to keep them from clamping shut
in a gesture of defense.

Even if the surgeon considers the procedure technically successful—in
that he was able to meet the goals that he set for himself and there were no
compromising complications—there is no way to know in the early days

and weeks postoperatively whether the surgery worked, whether its desired effect will actually be produced. That effect is, after all, not a property of the face itself but a response that the face will (hopefully) elicit. Such a measure of success cannot be clinically assessed nor known right away. Depending upon the procedures performed, it may take up to a year for all of the swelling to subside and for the face to "settle down," as surgeons say. Though new structures of bone and soft tissue were created in the event of the operation, the face itself is never a fixed and stable thing; it is always a thing unfolding in time, always seen anew by each person who encounters it.

After all of the waiting she has already done—waiting for self-acceptance, for surgery savings funds to grow, for consultations, for travel arrangements—now the surgical patient must wait to heal and find out whether the face she wanted is the face she's got. Surgery is the quintessential anticipatory regime (Adams et al. 2009). It is forward-looking, oriented to a future that will be meaningfully different from the life that would have unfolded without it. Surgery is intervention: the imagined and undesirable future can be changed by an operation. Once that event has occurred, there is nothing to do but wait. And hope.

This final chapter explores the "after" of FFS with the stories of three patients: Rachel was just recovering from surgery and was bursting with the optimism of a yet unknown future; Jill was ten years post-FFS and unreservedly happy with how the procedure had changed her life; and Zoe was three years post-FFS and disappointed that its promise of transformation had not been fulfilled. These three stories narrate the future not only of these three women but of American trans- medicine itself.

RACHEL

When I first met Rachel five days after her surgery I had to stifle a sympathetic wince. Her eyes were ringed in deep browns and purples, and the sutures beneath her nose drew contrastive attention to the thin red incision line where the length of her upper lip had been reduced. Though the packing had been removed from her nostrils earlier that day, the cast on her nose remained and was held in place by a large X of white tape rising up above her eyebrows and down across her cheeks. Her thinning hair and receding temporal baldness left sutures and staples visible across the crown of her head. I felt sore for her, as though neither of us should move too quickly. She, on the other hand, said she was feeling better than she had in days and was light on her feet as she offered me a tour of the Cocoon House, the private convalescent facility where she had been recovering.

The Cocoon House was a one-bedroom ground-floor apartment in a classic San Francisco two-flat building. It was owned and operated by an OR nurse who frequently worked with Ousterhout. She and her partner lived upstairs and helped provide support to FFS patients during their first days of recovery. The Cocoon House was affordable, located a short bus ride from Ousterhout's office, and was an important space of respite and camaraderie for patients who had traveled to San Francisco from other places. The bedroom and living room had both been converted into recovery spaces, each offering two beds so that patients' loved ones could stay with them. The apartment was not large, but it was well suited to recovery; there were no stairs to climb, and the pantry was stocked with single-serve containers of foods that were easy on a newly operated jaw: creamy soup, tomato juice, fruit cocktail, and chocolate pudding.

Following our short tour, Rachel led me to the back garden, where we could talk. As she spoke—with the marked accent and dry humor of a lifelong New Yorker—she dabbed saliva from the corners of her swollen mouth with a white cotton handkerchief. We talked for more than two hours with only one break: the unseasonably strong sun was heating the staples in her scalp and demanded that we move into the shade of a leafy tree.

Rachel, now in her mid-fifties, had first decided that she wanted FFS fifteen years earlier, as soon as she saw before-and-after photographs posted online: "From the moment I knew it existed, I thought, 'Wow.' I knew that I didn't have a pretty face. I'd get dressed up, but I knew I didn't look like a woman. I could put all the makeup in the world on and nobody was going to mistake me for a girl. Maybe when I was like sixteen. Essentially I would say that from the moment I knew people were doing it, I immediately started thinking to myself, 'Wow, I could do that too.'" When I asked her what it was about her face that she had wanted to change, she had trouble locating the problem she hoped surgery could fix—though she could quickly recount the list of the procedures that had just been performed. "If I was sitting here with a friend and just talking," she said, "I would say, 'Beauty is like pornography. You know it when you see it.' And it's the same thing with a feminine face: you know it when you see it." Though she noted that her "rather large nose" was "a male trait in [her] family," the nose by itself was not the problem. Neither, necessarily, was it her "fairly prominent forehead." It was something greater than these and something more diffuse.

I was a handsome man, but I didn't want to be handsome. I wanted to be pretty. I guess, in a certain sense, I wanted to have all the things that I enjoyed in women that I liked. The way they looked. The way their lips looked. What their hair looked like. How all the features went together. I think it's kind of a simple answer: I wanted to be a pretty girl. One of the great things that Dr. Ousterhout did was define this whole notion of feminizing in entirety, as opposed to just doing one thing. One thing in and of itself is not going to do it. It's got to be a holistic approach.

On account of her "holistic" transformation, Rachel did not really have an idea of what she would look like once her face had finished healing. More than any particular end point, what she most wanted her face to be was something other than what it had been for her entire adult life: masculine. The particular form her femininity would take did not concern her.

[When considering having FFS] I would say to [my friend], "Do I really want to do this? Because what if I don't really look good?" She would say to me, "Well, you know what you look like now. Would you rather go through the rest of your life looking like you look now, or looking like somebody else? Maybe you won't be drop-dead beautiful or even pretty, but you're not going to look like a man." So my answer was the latter. I knew how deeply dissatisfied I was. To the point of it being painful to look at myself in the mirror every day. That got worse as I got further into my transition. It just got worse and worse. The disconnect between what I felt and how I looked just became more and more pronounced, to the point where I just didn't want to look in the mirror. I just hated it. . . . [Someone] asked me, "Are you going to look very different [after FFS]?" And I said, "I sure hope so! That's the whole point." It wouldn't bother me if nobody recognized me. That wouldn't bother me at all. If somebody said, "You look fantastic, but I can't quite place you," that would be wonderful.

Under its bandages her new face—still tender, bruised, and cut—held the possibility of a radically new identity in which she could be a stranger to everyone she knew. That sounded scary to me, but to Rachel the prospect was "wonderful."

Rachel's personalized version of Ousterhout's early-morning doorbell scene recounted the promise of her total facial change:

My goal, my ideal is that I could go out on the street dressed like I'm dressed right now—just a pair of pants and a T-shirt and some sneakers—and no gender markings other than I'd be wearing earrings, which I always wear, and that when I went into a grocery store the person would say, "Can I help you, Miss?" That's really what I want. I want to be read as, accepted as, and reacted to as a woman. So that is what I was hoping [Ousterhout] would say he can do, and that's what he does say he can do. That *is* what he promises.

Becoming "accepted as and reacted to as a woman" would be the actualization of a truth about herself that Rachel traced back to her earliest childhood memories of dressing in her mother's lingerie and heels. Her knowledge of herself as being somehow "not right" had persisted throughout her life. "I've essentially been feeling ashamed of myself probably since I was four years old," she said. "Living daily with a sense of shame about who I was. And not only living with it but hiding it, because I was also hiding the source of my shame." She had undergone years of therapy with various psychologists and psychiatrists. When she was twenty a therapist told her there was no way to change the fundamentally feminine part of herself, but she couldn't accept that information then. "And out of everybody I saw in all the intervening years," she reflected, "what he said was the truth. It took me thirty years to accept that."

Rachel's feelings about herself as a trans- woman changed somewhat unexpectedly. Her mother was diagnosed with cancer, and as the child who lived closest, Rachel undertook what became a very intimate caretaking role during her mother's treatment. Despite long-standing conflicts in their relationship, many of which were rooted in Rachel's gender issues, the two grew close through this ordeal: "We were spending a lot of time together by ourselves. And I just sort of let go of any resentment or anger I had towards her, and I really just wanted to make her get well. Having a positive influence on her life kind of opened something in me that I had closed off. When the whole thing was over, I thought to myself, 'If I can give her this kind of love, then why can't I give it to myself?' So, I did." Tears streamed down her bruised cheeks as she recalled the epiphany that enabled her to accept herself as a trans- woman and also revived a loving relationship with her mother. "What started to happen for the first time in my life is that I started letting go of shame. I thought, 'I got my mother through this, how bad a person could I be? I *can't* be that bad.' So I started to just let go of feeling ashamed of myself, and feeling all this guilt. And that was a really new experience for me."

Her mother's cancer in remission and her divorce from her wife finalized, Rachel began hormone treatments, the beginning of her physical transition. "I had my first shot and it felt fantastic. I felt like Marilyn Monroe. I remember getting on the train going back downtown and I had to remind myself, 'You still look like a man to everybody.' That's how powerful it was. I recognize that it was psychological, but it was physical too."

Though she thought it was likely that she would eventually undergo genital sex-reassignment surgery and maybe breast augmentation, depending on how her breasts grew with hormone therapy alone, FFS was her first surgical priority. "The most important thing I could do was change my face," she explained. It was a change that would free her in ways that, on that sunny afternoon, she could only imagine.

Rachel's story bears common themes of many stories I heard. FFS was symbolic. It was climactic. It was the end of one story and poised as the beginning to another. Rachel didn't want to stop talking. She had so much to say. The procedure had been cathartic and made her wildly reflective on her whole life. She told me how she had fallen in and out of love with her former wife, about a long career in performing arts that she decided to leave behind, and about new hobbies and loves that she'd never tried before and was now exuberantly exploring. Her life was new since she decided to transition, and FFS was the first major actualization of this process—a step that was different, she explained, because unlike hormones, she couldn't take it back. For Rachel FFS was an act of self-love, and she was bursting.

Through word of mouth, personal experiences, and plenty of online research, Rachel, like most patients I met, felt confident that her wildest dreams could come true. She had seen scores of photographs of former FFS patients whose images and narratives of transformation attested to the possibility of total surgical transformation. It was the actualization of this idealized possibility that had earned Ousterhout a sort of cult following, and a legion of fans and defenders.

JILL

Ousterhout had performed Jill's full-face FFS nearly ten years before, and she had been an outspoken admirer and supporter of his ever since. "I've been a Doug girl for a long time," she said with a smile.

When I first met Jill, she reached into her pocket and pulled out her cell phone to show me a picture of what she looked like before surgery. I found the difference between the photograph and the face before me astounding. She clearly took great pride in this fact. "I don't reject who I was," she said of the man whose face she was showing me. "I don't apologize for what I was. I don't apologize for what I have become. I am comfortable with the unique mutt that I am, which is a combination of then and now. I like to think it's the best of both worlds as opposed to having to be one or the other." The photograph—and her narration of it—was an affirmation of her own reconciliation with her past and a testament to what FFS could do.

When Jill first learned about FFS in the late 1990s, she had already come to peace with the idea that she would never transition. She had a successful life as a husband and father and felt completely isolated in her knowledge of herself as a woman. If she could not be recognized by others as a woman, then she would have to learn to accept her life as it was. At that time, before the expansion of the Internet, she explained, "there was no validation. There was no hope that we could blend into society and just live our lives. The choices were twofold. One, you accept the fact that you live in the margins—if that was okay. Or you accept the fact that you live something less than a fulfilling life. I was married. I had a son. I had a good career. I had money. I had all of the trappings that society told me meant that I was successful, except that I had this secret." Jill described first learning that FFS was possible as a moment that was "very empowering, but it was also terrifying. When you become comfortable with the impossible, realizing that the impossible is possible gets scary."

Jill's initial surgery lasted nearly thirteen hours, and the recovery "was hell." Much like the radical transformation that Rachel envisioned, Jill's surgery had changed not only her face but her most basic understanding of herself and her world. Though she had not been politically engaged in her life as a man, since her transition—which began with FFS—Jill found herself confronted with social inequalities she had never been aware of before:

As a man I had never experienced discrimination. Really. Not that I knew of. You take it for granted: you're white, you're heterosexual—or perceived to be heterosexual—you're granted a level of privilege that you don't know that you have, that just comes with your birthright. You're living in a world that's oblivious to many of the unfortunate realities that others have to face. To have that stripped from you and see that people can be fired [for being trans-], people can lose their housing. To see that people in your community are not welcome in women's shelters but have too much self-respect to go to men's shelters and so they freeze to death on a park bench because they can't get a job and they're homeless. To recognize that in school people get the crap beat out of them because they're different. Those things are contrary to everything my parents raised me to believe. So I found that I was given opportunities to make choices.

Newly empowered by her changing body and newly outraged by an understanding of life she had not seen before, Jill became a prominent figure in trans- political organizing circles, delivering keynote addresses at national conferences and writing a widely circulated book about her experience of coming to terms with her identity and her process of transition. She attributed this radical shift in her life to FFS. "My own involvement never meant to be as significant as it became," she explained. "Going through this process was the single most profound experience of my entire life. It remains so. And I'll tell anybody who asks. The fact of the matter is that coming here, finally looking in the mirror and seeing somebody who more closely reflected on the outside who I knew I was on the inside and watching that person develop—because the person that I was six months after I left here was very different than the person who walked in here."

Jill was, quite literally, the poster girl for FFS and for Ousterhout. Her before-and-after photographs were featured in multiple places throughout Ousterhout's recently published book on FFS and were staples in his conference presentation slideshows. Not only did she epitomize the feminine—both visibly female and normatively beautiful—she also exemplified the total life-changing potential of FFS. Hers was a narrative of redemption that emphasized her own efforts for self-acceptance as materialized by Ousterhout, the person with the unique skills and vision to see in her—and make her into—the woman she knew herself to be.

Despite both her own and Ousterhout's characterization of her surgery as an unqualified success, Jill's time on the operating table was not done. She was in for some revision surgery on her jaw. In some patients the blood that pools around the bone following jaw-contouring surgery can later be reabsorbed and turn into bone. When this happened, patients often returned for revision in order to re-create the narrowed jaw that the initial surgery produced. This increasingly square jaw is what brought Jill back to the office. No face—no matter how fantastic—lasts forever.

ZOE

Not every patient had a surgical result and a story of triumph like Jill's. Zoe had decided that she wanted FFS early in her transition. "In terms of barriers to entry, the face is really important," she explained. "One's ability to be read as female really comes into play when deciding whether to transition. It's really difficult to be pegged as a trans-woman from twenty feet away. It was clear to me right away when I started cross-dressing that I would not pass as female without some work done on my face." Zoe had had a full-face FFS with Ousterhout nearly a year prior to our interview. She had returned to the office to consult with him about a repair to her nose (the structure of one nostril had collapsed, making it look pinched instead of round and open) and the possibility of re-raising her upper lip. (It was raised 3.5 millimeters in the initial surgery, but, like the squareness of Jill's jaw, the length of the upper lip can return over time.) These would have to wait, in any case, because paying for FFS and GSRS in the same year had left her on the verge of bankruptcy.

Zoe had initially been pleased with the results of her FFS. "Right after my surgery I passed really well, but lately I've had some really upsetting experiences." Though her FFS had certainly helped her to be recognized as a woman in casual exchanges, she found that the more time she spent with people, the greater the chance that their perception of her sex would change. This was particularly problematic because her work as an overseas flight attendant occasioned extended periods of time and (confined) interaction with new people. "I feel that working as a flight attendant is really empowering. I order people to sit down and fasten their seat belts, and they have to listen to me. There is a lot of power in this. On the other hand, sometimes the passengers torture me." Their comments and digs wore on her. "I do get read now," she explained, "but it happens gradually. Like, if I'm in a flight it won't happen for ten or fifteen minutes." After that time passengers had ways of letting her know they were reading her as a transwoman. "They'll call me 'ma'am' when they get on the plane, but 'sir' when they get off," she said. "Or someone will start to whistle 'For He's a Jolly Good Fellow' and I turn around and they stop. I can't tell who's doing it.

In these situations you really feel the hostility of straight people." Her face and neck grew red as she recounted these cutting and infantile exchanges.

Zoe explained that in spite of the feminizing effects of hormones and the fact that she had DD-size breasts, her face continued to mark her as trans-. She told me her face frequently drew unwelcome attention, making even a trip to the pharmacy to buy cough syrup a humiliating and self-scrutinizing event.

A few days ago I was in Walgreens and a guy turns around and says, "You're hot. I saw you in Starbucks yesterday. My friend and I are wondering if you're a man." I said, "You're staring at my breasts, you tell me." He said, "I think you're hot, but my friend thinks you're a dude." Even though I know I shouldn't care about stupid shit like this, it really hurts me. I wanted FFS in order to avoid these kinds of situations. I know this surgery doesn't come with a guarantee that no one will call you a man again, but I feel like that was happening for six months. But for the past six months it isn't anymore.

A few weeks before our interview armed guards pulled Zoe out of the security checkpoint line in the Dubai Airport. The officers took her into a small room and asked her point blank if she was a man. "I said no. He asked to see my passport, which says *Female*, and he still didn't believe me. I thought, 'Oh, fuck. What do I do now?'" Suspecting that she was male, the guard informed her that there was a penalty for lying about gender in the United Arab Emirates. "Eventually I told him that he could see my vagina if he didn't believe me. Thank god I had one. That must have pushed him over the line because he just let me go." Zoe wiped tears from her eyes. "It was terrifying."

Despite the fact that she was still sometimes read as male, Zoe credited FFS with having saved her life. As long as her social interactions were brief and "casual," she was recognized as a woman. It was a welcome, if fleeting, reprieve.

I felt that FFS was a necessary part of my transition because I had to avoid looking like a cross-dressed male. Therapists have said to me that there is nothing to do but be yourself. But for trans- people I think that is really disingenuous. Surgery is what enables me to physically and psychically be myself. I'm the only forty-five-year-old woman I know who jumps out of bed in the morning to look at my naked body and feels like cheering. That wouldn't be possible without surgery. [FFS] saved me from suicide. It gave me the ability to have a life, to function. I used to spend hours on my hair and makeup, but I always looked like a cross-dressed male. For six months post-op I wasn't a circus act or the center of attention. That's not really working anymore, but casually my life is better. I just can't deal with the shit every day.

Zoe was obviously disappointed. She had hoped that her story would end the way Jill's had, that FFS would actualize her fantasy of being unquestionably recognized as a woman in all situations. But it wasn't working out that way. Despite extensive facial reconstruction at the cost of many thousands of dollars—and surgical breast augmentation and an ongoing regimen of hormone replacement and body hair removal—she was still being recognized as a trans- woman and suffering the very real consequences that often came with it.

WHAT DO I LOOK LIKE?

Zoe was among a small minority of Ousterhout's FFS patients who were unhappy with their results. Her stories about the airport, the pharmacy, and the plane passengers were offered as proof that the promise of FFS had not been met, that the surgery hadn't worked. Ousterhout didn't see it that way. Zoe's stories meant something else to him. Because Ousterhout believed the certainty of the female face is total, the suggestion that a person's *face* could be recognized as male following a full-face FFS operation simply made no sense. As such, the problem must not be her face; the problem was either that she was misperceiving others' responses to her postoperative face or that she was failing to make other parts of her body signify femaleness as strongly as her newly rebuilt face did.

In general Ousterhout believed that when patients reported they were still being recognized as trans- women after a full-face FFS, they were simply misinterpreting the looks and responses of others:

> I think what happens with a lot of people is that for so many years people look at you. You're dressed as a female, you haven't had any surgery, and you become rather paranoid. Maybe there's a better word. But people look at you and say, "There's obviously a transsexual." But then [after FFS], when you start looking good as a female, people

look at you and you have a tendency to think the same thing [as be-fore]. You say, "They're reading me [as trans-]." They're not. They're admiring you. They're looking at you like you're an attractive woman.

It may be that none of us is ever quite sure why another person is looking at us, but in his telling the only person who *does* know why a trans- woman is the object of another's gaze is her surgeon.

Like all patients, when Zoe first came to consult about the possibility of FFS, her experiences of being seen by others as trans- were substantiated by her surgeon's identification of her masculine features. In this process her experience of her body's masculinity was externalized, reified, and verified by medical authority. Before surgery, the surgeon acknowledged that Zoe knew why people were looking at her, and he agreed with her assessment that her face's problematic masculinity was visible to others. After surgery, however, the knowledge produced by Zoe's experience of being recognized as trans- did not have the same value. Ousterhout interpreted Zoe's ex-change at the airport as the result of her postoperative good looks. In his version of the story the guards were not reading Zoe as trans-; they were "letches" who wanted to "mess with a pretty girl" because "they're not get-ting any at home." Harassment and objectification were simply aspects of being a beautiful woman to which Zoe had yet to adapt. More than that, the attention from these guards proved to Ousterhout that Zoe's surgery had been a success. If she were not beautiful, he reasoned, the guards would never have bothered her. He was certain Zoe was misguided in interpreting the airport event as confirmation that her FFS had not worked. He saw her version of the story as evidence of an unfortunate and paranoiac inability to understand how and as what other people saw her. Because she had been the object of negative attention for so long, he suggested, she no longer knew how to recognize attention when it was positive; she didn't under-stand what she looked like.

Zoe knew that her dissension made her a "difficult patient." "Dr. Ouster-hout immediately called Mira in when he saw that I was going to be a com-plex appointment," she told me. "Now I have to deal with her in order to get to him. It's frustrating. He doesn't like my complaints." Zoe felt powerless. Her FFS did not do for her what she hoped it would do. Ousterhout, who, prior to surgery, was among the only people who could "see" her feminine face beneath her masculine one, now utterly dismissed the notion that any masculinity remained.

Ousterhout determined that Zoe's postsurgical symptoms—her experiences of being read and reacted to as a trans- woman—had no clinical basis. Whereas before her surgery Ousterhout and Zoe agreed about the masculine properties of her face, now they disagreed about what her face looked like. In such a situation patients' opinions are often dismissed in favor of surgical authority (Lorber 1975; Pitts-Taylor 2007; Plemons 2015). "Where the surgeon deems the operation a success," Suzanne Fraser (2003:126) writes, "the patient's failure to agree is pathologised." Instead of evidence to the contrary, Zoe's persistent assertions that she was being recognized as trans- functioned to undermine her credibility as a reasonable person and a good patient. It also marked her as a typically difficult trans- patient, a figure that has populated clinical literature since the 1950s (Habal 1990; Lothstein 1979; van de Ven 2008). The "problem patient" is a concern in all aesthetic and reconstructive surgery as patients and surgeons work to differently balance the promise that surgery can be transformative, but only up to a point. The assessment of surgical outcomes privileges a surgeon's professional expertise above the experience of the patient who lives in the altered body. "Due to the subjective quality of judgments about aesthetic appeal," Fraser (2003:127) writes, "surgeons are in a somewhat unique position to argue that the results of their surgery are successful even when the participant does not agree. In fact, participants' disagreement on this point is sometimes posed as an indicator of mental disability *in itself*."

The claim that animates FFS—that surgeons can create a feminine face that everyone will see as female and thus render patients recognizable as women—is quite grand in scale. In surgical discourse the idea that sex and gender can be totally transformed is "realistic," but any idea on behalf of patients about the precise form that transformation will take—even ideas expressly encouraged by surgeons—can be resignified after the surgery as unrealistic and characteristic of a constitutively pathological demand (Plemons 2015). In these cases it is the surgeon and his team who are at risk of burning out and buckling under the stress of the expectations of transformation that the surgical team helped to cultivate.

A Belgian FFS surgeon, Bart van de Ven (2008:294), cautions surgeons to be aware of what makes their trans- patients distinct and potentially problematic: "In most aesthetic operations, patients would like to improve their looks but above all continue to look like themselves. When it comes to facial feminisation, patients wish to change dramatically. This means it is easy for patients to develop unrealistic expectations. Some even come with photos of other women that they would like to resemble. As a surgeon, it is very important to make clear to the patient that you will do your best to make her as feminine as possible, but you cannot change her into another woman." I would argue, however, that "changing her into another woman" is precisely what animates the promise of FFS. It is what Rachel hoped for in being unrecognizable to her friends, what Jill got when she left her quotidian life as a husband and became a sought-after political activist, and what Zoe mourned when the scorn she experienced as a trans- woman remained at the cost of her best efforts and her life savings.

FFS is a project committed to creating "woman" as a socially recognizable category and in that sense is a project of ontological invention. As such, changing the patient from an unrecognizable woman into a recognizable woman is exactly what Ousterhout and Beck promise to do. The preoperative patient is one whose status as a woman is hers alone to assert, often in direct and painful contrast to the perceptions and attributions of others. The postoperative woman is (ideally) one whose status as a woman is reflected by and thus given iteratively by those around her. It is the desire to change from one to the other that motivates patients to seek out and undergo this change.

In cases like Zoe's, where FFS fails to live up to its promise of certain and enduring femaleness, the patient and the surgeon inevitably locate the fault of this failure differently. For the surgeon the issue is located either firmly in the misdirected mind of the patient or spread out across her entire body—to everywhere except her face. The preoperative promise that facial surgery can totally change a patient's social body is completely forgotten when patients return to the clinic unhappy with their results. Now, doctors acknowledge, sex and gender markers are everywhere: vocal pitch, patterns of speech, dress, hair, makeup, and on and on. Since her face simply cannot be the problem, it must be something else. It is up to the patient to "pile on" the signifiers, to support her changed face by learning to dress like, walk like, talk like, and otherwise effect *woman*. While the preoperative fantasy is that the face will change everything, after surgery the face can do only so much. The doctor can do only what he can do. Zoe had met the limit of what (this) surgery could do for her.

Despite the disappointment and increasing despair that came from her depleted emotional and financial resources, Zoe continued her efforts to cultivate a recognizable femaleness through the deployment of new bodily strategies:

> I have found that the way I choose to dress myself has the biggest impact on passing or not. Dressing to expose my breasts just makes my life easier. [She pointed at the low-cut sweater and lacy camisole she was wearing.] It is a choice between being read as a cross-dressed male or a strange-looking, slutty woman. Women are much less nice when I have the cleavage from my DDs showing, but men are infinitely kinder, gentler, and more attentive. When I cover my breasts and rely on my face and body to gender me, men are cruel. Someone yelled "Hey, amigo!" at me on the street the other day. I am harassed and not taken seriously when I show my breasts, but I don't get brought to tears for looking slutty.

Though she made it clear that her preference would have been to dress more conservatively, Zoe had found that she had to work with the sex and gender markers that worked for her. This decision cost her something she had not intended to lose. She was seen as a woman only when she was a *kind* of woman she didn't want to be. Being seen as a "strange-looking, slutty woman" was preferable to being seen as a "cross-dressed male"; nevertheless it was a compromise beyond the momentous morning doorbell scene that anchored the promise of FFS. Her new face, as it turned out, was not the key to the radically reconfigured life she'd hoped for. Instead she had to keep working—both with and around her face and body—to get from others the recognition she longed for. Yet she hadn't given up on the promise of FFS. Her faith that Ousterhout could do something more, that facial reconstruction was still the answer, had brought her back to ask for revisions.

For trans- women, as for all women, femininity is a receding horizon. The feminine body requires constant maintenance and vigilance against time, its perpetual enemy. Patients often fantasized that the day of the operation would mark the date when the problem of their masculine face—and thus the attribution of maleness by others—would be gone forever. This fantasy freezes time and is made possible, in part, by a discourse of "the female" that is itself context-free and timeless. But every fantasy is negated in the act of its production; no face can be as good in real life as was the surgical panacea of the imagination. Aging patients learned that the fantasy of a now and forever femininity cannot hold. Zoe was certainly not the only FFS patient to find herself back in the chair, hoping for surgical revisions. Even those like Jill who were happy with their results often came back for facelifts and touch-ups years down the road as they learned, like all women, that femininity is always on the wane.

CONCLUSION

There is no single answer to the question of whether FFS works and, if it does, what kinds of work it does. In the end the question of its efficacy, of whether FFS does what it promises to do, is not a question of the technical or the surgical. This is because, as Ousterhout's denial of Zoe's experience makes clear, the sex/gender of a face is not only a property of the face itself. The face is the primary site of our individuality and bodily identity, and the dynamism and ultimate effect of FFS is produced through interaction.

Readers have likely noticed that there are no photographs of FFS patients in this book. When I first began presenting this work people often asked to see before-and-after photographs, and at first I indulged their requests. Curious viewers wanted to know if the transformation FFS promised could actually take place, if there was some surgical means of changing their perceptions of something so basic about a person as their sex. Some viewers remarked on the startling changes they saw. They marveled at the surgical capability manifest in the images and typically included a simultaneous incredulous and laudatory claim along the lines of "Wow, I would ne' know that she was trans-!" Others would criticize and undermine the fectiveness of the surgeries by claiming the opposite: "I can totally tel' was a man." In both cases the respondents were expressing wheth' had *worked on them*. The project and promise of FFS is, of course, n' happens to the viewer when FFS works but what happens to th' woman herself.

Knowing in advance that what they were seeing was the facia' mation of trans- women who had undergone FFS, viewers w'ity assess their own abilities and limitations in recognizing facia'ame (for it is masculinity that is visible when one "can still tell"). ny FFS clear to me in witnessing these assessments is a realization patients lived with every day: once performed, FFS cannot be said simply to have "worked" or "not worked." Such an assessment, like the attribution of sex/gender in general, depends on who is looking and what they're looking for. By not including before-and-after photos I hope to make clear that whether or not you, dear reader, are able to see a trans- woman in the context of a book about trans- women is totally irrelevant. The aim of these surgical interventions is invisible femininity, the kind you don't look at twice. I can show you neither what that is nor what it is not. Instead I've let the patients and surgeons tell you what it is for them as they work to enact it with all of our viewing and assessing eyes in mind.

In the introduction I posed two questions: How did the claim that a person could change sex through facial surgery come to acquire a rhetoric of common sense in the mid-1990s? What can the growing popularity of FFS tell us about the changing practices of trans- medicine and the concepts of sex and gender on which it depends? This book has tried to answer these questions. Let me remind you how.

First, a trans- patient treated under the midcentury model of genital-centric transsexual medicine found that her genital surgery did not produce the change in social identity that she longed for. Her desire to be accepted and recognized as a woman—not only to have the genital structure of a female—prompted the search for a distinctly female skull that could guide surgical practice. This was not a disinterested scientific search for the truth of human forms. It was, like all scientific and medical endeavors, informed by existing values. In this case those included a collapse between the biology of female bodies and the desirability of feminine beauty, and an uncritical reliance on and reproduction of whiteness as the unmarked and ideal feminine bodily form. The emergence of this model became a touchstone that both technically enabled and ethically justified the growing practice of FFS by the mid-1980s.

FFS didn't grow in popularity merely because it was surgically possible. A changing political and economic landscape in the United States beginning the 1990s contributed to an exponential expansion of elective surgery in eral and a new attitude toward trans- medicine in particular. Beck's case onstrated how the move away from paternalistic gender clinics in the and toward market medicine in the 1990s corresponded with a new e of trans- medicine. No longer treatment for a "wrong body" dis-a ns- surgery could be, like surgery for millions of other Americans, ward individual authenticity and self-actualization. The binary model of the body that guided an either/or approach to surgical sex reassignment could be replaced by a "real me" intervention, aiming not to make stable male and female bodies but to make authentic identities visible.

In spite of market expansion and a new discourse of self-actualization, medical attitudes toward trans- people have been slow to change. As such, the emotional work done in surgical clinics was vital to the success of FFS. In contrast to harmful or resistant doctors who punished or willing doctors who pitied, contemporary trans- surgeons wielded beneficent compassion as itself a surgical technique. This was crucial for patients as they looked for surgeons who could actualize their fantasies of enduring and permanent womanhood. By reproducing trans- narratives, offering themselves as "friends to the community," and cultivating a staff of affirming and supportive listeners, surgeons made FFS work as an act of restitutive intimacy, framing technical work in the surgical present as means to right injustices in the surgical past.

It is as a result of these confluences that FFS acquired a rhetoric of self-evidence in the mid-1990s: a surgical claim that faces could be made distinctly sexed was incorporated into trans- medicine; there was an expanded market of self-actualization that corresponded with the emergence of performative claims to sex/gender as a product of social recognition; and there was a growing group of trained surgeons and staff willing to commit to the efficacy of FFS as a life- and sex-changing technology.

The proliferation of treatment modalities employed in trans- medicine is making new demands on the ways that effects of treatment interventions are understood, and thus what comes to be legible as good trans- medicine. No longer limited to a story of individual transformation, the expansion of recognition-based understandings of sex and gender and the collapse between them (sex/gender) are powerfully bringing the body's social life into focus and, in the process, revealing fractures and fissures that a limited focus on passing can obscure. Conflicting terms of recognition—at the level of the collective and as registered by the state—demonstrate a proliferation of competing terms, concepts, and ways of understanding what trans- medicine can and should do. Instead of a paradigm shift, in which one approach to understanding and medically responding to trans- people's request for surgery completely replaces another, ideas and responses are multiplying, sometimes in ways that render them illegible to each other. Passing is neither the undisputed goal of trans- medicine nor an adequate analytic with which to understand all of its effects. The subject of trans- therapeutics is no longer atomistic; it is tied to collective projects of political justice and compels legal and policy engagement from the state in a number of ways. As demands for trans- health care and insurance coverage continue to expand, this dynamic scene will continue to unfold.

In spite of the unsettled, multiple, and contested scenes in which the practice of American FFS unfolds, there is a material urgency to surgery. In the operating room, where bones are sawed and burred and skin is excised and discarded, the openness of interpretation recedes to the background and the constrained act of physical transformation moves to the fore. In this scene the aspirational aim of recognition is confronted with the body's material limits. This materiality both invites and pushes back on the performative logic that underwrites FFS. We can see the prescriptive interventions in FFS as the effect of norming powers that narrowly define who may be counted in the category woman, and we can also see that reproducing expectations is the surest way to be counted there. Being counted as women was the deep and sincere goal that animated patients' hopes for FFS and directed surgeons' treatment plans. Claims that recognition is the means through which legible forms of personhood are enacted can sometimes contend less with the historicity of norms than with the pressing need of the present. Descriptions of Rosalind's surgery demonstrated this tension, showing how, as a discursive resource, performativity enables a critical analysis of FFS at the same time that it produces and authorizes a surgical plan for its success. It is in their ability to jar sex/gender out of individual genital anatomies and put it into historically particular understandings of bodies and selves as effects of collective life that have made recognition-based theories so powerful and transformative.

And still recognition is less certain as a measure of identity than are discrete anatomical forms. Hopes for and effects of FFS, located as they are in the imagined and actual responses of others, are fragile things. Others can refuse to recognize. They can punish. They can deny. They can transform the body from a site of hopeful possibility into a seemingly immovable blockade of flesh and bone. Whether FFS works is determined by the life of the face as a social thing, not a discrete and atomized anatomy. Perceptions give sense to the body; they give its matter meaning. The ways a face—or any other body part—acts to either facilitate or limit the possibility of a recognizable sex/gender is not static. It does not reflect the stability of a dimorphic skeleton or simply reflect back the qualities of a celebrity headshot. There is no specific thing here, no single female face, no one formula for a womanhood that will be recognized by all. FFS is the physical manifestation of a particular way of understanding what a woman is. Its enactments include the participation of an ever-rotating audience, an unending crowd who will recognize a trans- woman's womanhood. Or not.

FFS exemplifies the changing aims and conceptual underpinnings of trans- medicine; it materializes a trans- therapeutics centered on sex as an effect of everyday interaction. This kind of bodily sex is not focused inward, to the body's concealed properties, concealed under clothing or within hormones or chromosomes; it is focused outward, to the constitution of "real" sex as a fact of lived reality. Thus it is a model of sex change aimed at changing recognition more than any particular anatomical feature. FFS is about creating in the body of the patient the expectations of the audience, about making a face that others will respond to and treat as the face of a woman.

I have treated the performative logic of sex/gender as an ethnographic fact to show how the emergence of this way of thinking about sex/gender has become a discursive resource, a means for understanding and explaining trans- body projects as oriented to a kind of sex that was not centered on genitals and did not depend on essential claims to permanence. Recognition-based formulations of sex and of sex change have been adopted into medical practice, in part, by the fact that when university clinics closed in the 1980s, trans- folks with financial resources left the role of patient-recipient and began directing their transitions as patient-clients. Alongside the development and popularization of performative means of thinking sex/gender, American medicine changed considerably in the 1990s, ushering in a new relationship to surgical body projects. These two factors helped to support the growth of trans- political movements in America that explicitly rejected the essentialist framework within with the diagnosis of transsexualism and its genital-centric treatments had been organized. There were new choices for transition and new ways to define what patients wanted from it.

FFS is a set of practices guided by history, by markets, by expertise, and by charisma. It is an example of how ideas about how to define sex, gender, and transgender, man, woman, and everything between, get written into the medical practices aimed at instantiating members of those categories. Like all forms of trans- medicine, FFS materializes *man, woman, male,* and *female* into action. It incites a logic of trans- therapeutics into speech, makes a claim about why, how, and toward what ends trans- people seek medicosurgical interventions, and designs interventions in spite of uncertain definitions. In the FFS clinical office patients and surgeons assert a trans- therapeutics centered on a body enlivened and invested with socially particular meanings. They enact a surgical logic that moves sex/gender out of individual bodies and into the social space between people, where the performative claim that sex/gender is made real through recognition can be worked into a surgical plan.

As Rachel and I sat talking in that back garden, she told me she didn't really have a sense of what she would look like when all the sutures were removed and all the bruises faded away. She'd done her homework, and then she'd picked a surgeon and deferred to his expertise to do the things that must be done. She didn't particularly care how she looked, as long as the surgery worked. If it did, she didn't particularly care how or why it did. "How many times have people told me in the last year how brave I am? And I appreciate it that they say it, but I really don't look at it that way. It's only brave because people make it so hard. You know, if somebody sets your house on fire, is it brave to run out of it? That's how I see it. I'm running out of a burning house at this point. I guess I could have just sat there and died. I changed my face so that I could run out."

There was no way to know what might happen some Saturday morning, when she walked into the grocery store and turned her face to the checkout clerk. No way to know what the clerk would see, or what they would say. All there was to do was sit and wait.

NOTES

INTRODUCTION

1 Sex and gender identities and terminologies proliferate. In recent years the word *transgender* has become common as an umbrella term meant to encompass a wide variety of established and emerging identities. This language is constantly shifting and being inhabited differently by different people. When I write about trans- people as a larger group, I adopt the term *trans-*. Whereas Stryker et al. (2008) use the term *trans-* in order to leave open the possibility of kinds of crossing that are not limited to gender, I use the open-ended hyphen to call attention to the many possible endings of the term, all of which are important to the people who identify themselves as such.

2 U.S. Department of Health and Human Services, "Nondiscrimination in Health Programs and Activities," 81 Fed. Reg. 96 (May 18, 2016), *Federal Register: The Daily Journal of the United States*, July 2016. Online.

3 Drs. Ousterhout and Joel Beck insisted that I identify them by their real names. All other names of patients and doctors are pseudonyms, except those cited in published works.

4 For early European clinical trials on FFS, see Becking et al. 1996; Gooren and Doorn 1997; Hage et al. 1997a, 1997b. For invocations of eventual FFS as an endorsement of adolescent hormone intervention, see Cohen-Kettenis et al. 2008, 2011; Rosenthal 2014; Shumer and Spack 2013. For a critical discussion of such endorsements, see Sadjadi 2013.

5 Butler's contemporaries who were taking up the gendered histories of sciences in other terms include Jordanova 1989; Laqueur 1990; Russett 1989; Schiebinger 1989, 1993; Stepan 1986.

6 Of course credit for this shift in thinking about gender does not go to Butler alone. One could call on a long tradition of sociology, from Cooley to Goffman and later Garfinkle (1967) and Kessler and McKenna (1978), who have all studied gender as a form of socially structured doing, a deliberate action that gets its sense through recognition. Anthropological scholarship of gender has had an abiding interest in attending to specific social practices and how they trouble simple biological narratives of sex difference. These stretch back to Margaret Mead ([1935] 2001) and Ruth Benedict

(1939) and, more influential in the latter twentieth century's development of gender theory, to the pathbreaking work of Esther Newton (1972, 2000; see Rubin 2002). Butler's crucial contribution to these long and fruitful lines of scholarship was to use the critical lens of gender enactment to destabilize the givenness of sex.

7　By the end of the 1990s the theory of gender performativity had traveled far beyond the readers of Butler's abstruse text. By the time *Gender Trouble*'s tenth anniversary edition was published in 1999, claims to performative sex/gender had been explicitly invoked by activists, used by the American Psychoanalytic Association and the American Psychological Association to reassess their principles and positions on homosexuality, engaged in art exhibits at prestigious galleries, and used in jurisprudence and legal scholarship (Butler 1999:xvii). In 2001 the *International Journal of Sexuality and Gender Studies* published a double issue on Butler's impact on fields as diverse as archaeology, film, Renaissance studies, and political theory. Butler's work on sex/gender in the 1990s helped mark a fundamental shift in the way many people understand what sex and gender are, how they are done, and how they might be productively done otherwise (see Schippers 2014:1). Stripped of the intricate conceptual links in which Butler had suspended it, decontextualized from its long and rich histories in linguistic scholarship (see Bauman and Briggs 1990), *performativity* became a metonymic shorthand for a bold new response to the constraints of essentialist and biologically centered theories of sex and gender against which feminist and social constructionist thinkers had been agitating in the 1970s and 1980s. Condensing meanings beyond those Butler initially assigned it, gender performativity became a discursive resource—a distinct way of thinking and talking about subjects and bodies, knowledge and power—by which new claims to the nature of sex and gender could be made.

8　Statistics kept on the incidence of cosmetic and reconstructive surgeries show an increase in these procedures and dollars spent on them year over year since professional groups began collecting these data in the mid-1990s (ASAPS 1997; ASPS 2014).

9　Still others argue that the goal of passing can obscure and effectively foreclose the possibility of a trans- specific radical political subjectivity (Bornstein 1994; Green 1999; Stone [1991] 2006). This group does not object to passing per se; they are concerned with what strategies of erasing trans- visibility mean to a liberatory politics premised on making space for difference by rendering difference visible. For a history of the prefix *cis-* as applied to gender and sex, see Aultman 2014; Enke 2013.

10　For critiques of Taylor and Honneth on this point, see McBride 2013; McQueen 2015.

11　It's not uncommon for trans- people to experience "research fatigue" (Davidmann 2014:110), the exhaustion of being asked over and over again to contribute to research studies. I was acutely aware of this risk, especially since much of my research took place inside the especially vulnerable space of the surgeon's office. The presence of an observer inevitably impacts the clinical dynamic. I tried to minimize my impact on clinical interactions by remaining outside the patient's field of vision whenever possible, by giving patients the option to include me in some clinical interactions but exclude me from others, and by reserving questions and discussion with the surgeon not only to times away from patients, but when there were no patients in the office. Still, there is no disappearing as the third party to a two-person exchange. Sometimes surgeons used my face as an example to describe characteristics. Sometimes patients wanted or felt compelled to talk with me in the lulled and anxious minutes waiting for the surgeon to return to the consultation room. Sometimes they asked me questions about their own consultation, knowing that I had observed several others and that I had experiences that were from the perspective of neither patient nor doctor. In these ways, I became a part of the clinical experience for patients, a resource for reflection or for information.

My one-on-one interviews with patients (I conducted twenty-eight formal interviews) frequently took place in a side office in the clinic, but sometimes patients preferred to meet elsewhere, including the hospital cafeteria or the convalescent facility, or to talk while walking in a park near the hospital. Not all those I asked to participate in this research agreed to take part. Some declined completely. A few consented to allow me to observe in the operating room once they were under anesthesia but did not want to talk with me. Out of respect for patients, adherence to research protocols, and deference to the principles of anthropological scholarship, I deferred to participants' wishes and allowed those who did want to talk with me to set the tone and length of our interaction. Some formal interviews lasted just fifteen minutes; others lasted for more than two hours.

Disclosing the fact that I am trans- was sometimes helpful in building rapport with the trans- women I talked with. In some instances it helped to produce a kind of fellow feeling and assured my interlocutors that I was not interested in pathologizing or exoticizing them, as so much research has done. Nor was I interested in turning their stories into melodramatic tales of suffering or hagiographic tales of resilience. My trans- status also became a tool for conversation. For example, a patient named Rhonda described knowing she was a woman "ever since [she] came out of her mother's womb," and then stopped and said, "Well, *you* know what I mean!" Her assumption about our common experience allowed her to share and relate to me as an insider.

That there was a significant gap between my story of medical transition and theirs was a fact not lost on the trans- women with whom I spoke during my fieldwork. Trans- women often remarked at how masculine I was. They looked me up and down and asked how long I had been on testosterone. I was once called a "lucky son of a bitch." Though I had found these kinds of comments irksome (because they made me self-conscious and were too often accompanied by what felt like condescending squeezes of my biceps), in the course of this project I have come to understand them differently.

I · On Origins

1   For more on the founding and activities of the Erickson Educational Foundation, see Devor 2002; Devor and Matte 2004, 2007.
2   Documenting the existence and operations of these clinics is a difficult task. In addition to the officially and institutionally recognized centers counted by Restack

(1979), a number of other gender clinics—or clinics providing transition-related services—were operating in the United States in the 1960s and 1970s. One example is the University of Michigan. University archives date the existence of their gender program to 1993, but I interviewed professionals associated with a consistent program of trans- related care that began in 1968. Documenting this history is vital not only for the enrichment of trans- and medical history but also to inform a new generation of university-based American clinics that have begun to emerge following the 2014 changes in Medicare and other insurance policies.

3   In addition to losing surgeons, university-based clinics were also losing funding as the Erickson Educational Foundation began to direct its philanthropic dollars elsewhere (Devor and Matte 2007). The diagnosis of transsexualism appeared in the American Psychiatric Association's *Diagnostic and Statistical Manual (III-R)* for the first time in 1980, which, along with the creation of the first clinical Standards of Care for "the hormonal and surgical sex reassignment of gender dysphoric persons" (Harry Benjamin International Gender Dysphoria Association 1979) effectively decentralized evaluation and diagnosis from the university clinics to any mental health care provider who was willing to apply the relevant criterion (Stryker 1999). Even more damning was the publication of a 1979 research study arguing that genital sex-reassignment surgery conferred no measurably therapeutic benefit to patients (Meyer and Reter 1979). Contested though it was, the study dealt a critical blow to clinics whose existence was already embroiled in controversy and threatened by financial challenges (Rudacille 2005).

4   This designation indicates a combined specialty. A maxillofacial surgeon works on the entire skull and face, including the upper and lower jaws. Craniofacial surgery is a subspecialty of maxillofacial surgery that typically addresses congenital deformities of the skull, face, and jaw.

5   Aleš Hrdlička is widely acknowledged as the founding figure of American physical anthropology. He founded the *American Journal of Physical Anthropology* in 1918 and served a forty-year tenure as the curator of the Division of Physical Anthropology at the American Museum of Natural History (later the Smithsonian Institute) beginning in 1903. During this time Hrdlička amassed what was then the largest collection of human osteological material in the world (Hrdlička 1919; Montagu 1944).

6   Although interrogation of received wisdom about sexual difference emerged in archaeological scholarship alongside the analytical concept of gender, in recent years archaeologists have taken up the tools of queer theory to trouble sex/gender dichotomies. See Geller 2005, 2008, 2016; Gere 1999; Joyce 2005, 2008; Sofaer 2006. For an excellent review of this literature, see Ghisleni et al. 2016.

7   On the concept of population, see Haraway 1997:248–49; Haraway 1989:212–14.

8   In the first surgical publication to describe the morphological characteristics of skulls with the express purpose of transforming their sexed distinctions, Ousterhout (1987) cited six sources for his claim to anthropological distinctions between male and female skulls: a book on forensic anthropology that identified aspects of the face frequently used to assign sex (Stewart 1979); an article on the utility of facial modeling to identify the dead based on skeletal remains (Snow et al. 1970);

and four articles on the use of a statistical operation called discriminant function analysis to determine sex based on skeletal materials, mostly mandibles (Giles 1964; Giles and Elliot 1963; Stewart 1954; Thieme and Schull 1957).

9 For the purposes of the study, *normal* meant only that students were enrolled in the mainstream school and did not assume any representativeness of the population.

10 The USGS and ten of the eleven known collections of longitudinal growth materials in the United States and Canada together form the American Association of Orthodontists Foundation Craniofacial Growth Legacy Collection.

11 The unmarked whiteness of the normal form presented in the USGS *Atlas* reflects the absence of concern for racial difference, although many contemporary orthodontic researchers were interested in morphological differences based on race. A few small cephalometric studies were done to assess racial difference in the later twentieth century (Alexander and Hitchcock 1978; Altemus 1960; Drummond 1968; Richardson 1980). For an early discussion of the problem of applying "the white standards" to other groups, see Cotton et al. 1951.

12 Through his own efforts and those of an extended network of friends and colleagues, Atkinson's collection included skulls from Africa, Australia, Japan, and China and of native peoples from North, Central, and South America (Pollock 1969). According to a 1969 article by H. C. Pollock, "Indian examples from the West Coast of North America are included, as well as those of the Flathead Indians of Montana and the Pueblo Indians of New Mexico" (511). Atkinson himself "searched and unearthed several Indian mounds in California and on the islands off the California coast" (512). According to Dorothy Dechant, the collection includes fifteen skulls from Native Americans, an unusually small number for an American collection. Due to the ethical and political complications of holding Native American remains since the 1990 passage of the Native American Graves Protection and Repatriation Act, Dechant does not acquire or accept donations of Native American remains for the collection. She reported that she had not encountered any conflict over repatriation in relation to the library's existing holdings.

13 This is considered by many researchers to be a significant shortcoming of the collection, and is a main reason the collection is used by only about ten researchers each year.

14 As part of the original research that produced FFS, Ousterhout (1987) developed a typological scheme that both described male foreheads and indicated the surgical techniques necessary to bring them into the proportions of the female norm. He referred to these as forehead types I, II, III, and IV.

15 On the emergence of *transgender*, see Califia 1997; Meyerowitz 2002; Roebuck 2013; Stryker 2008; Valentine 2007.

INTERLUDE. *The Procedures*

1 One American FFS surgeon claims that he can produce all of the same bone restructuring results through endoscopy. In my conversations with other surgeons, this claim was hotly disputed.

1   The issue for which trans- people seek medical intervention has been theorized as an endocrine imbalance, a psychoanalytic failure of proper identification, a genetic defect, a morphological defect, a failure of imprinting, and an indication of profound delusional psychopathology. Elsewhere it has been criminal, antisocial, antifeminist, and indicative of a sinister deceitfulness (Cohen-Kettenis and Gooren 1999; Daly 1978; Gooren 2006; Hausman 1995; Hoenig 1985; Jeffreys 2014; Lothstein 1982; Raymond 1979).

2   This is especially true in the context of American medicine, in which patients coordinate their own transition-related care, carting copies of their own diagnostic documents across town or across the country to seek care from mental health, medical, and surgical practitioners who in all likelihood will never personally interact. Though the Standards of Care recommended by the World Professional Association for Transgender Health advocate coordinated care among clinicians with different specialties, such teams are rare in the United States.

3   For a critique of such use of anthropological examples, one that they call "romancing the transgender native," see Towle and Morgan 2002.

4   This essay was first published on the website *GenderTalk* in 1995. It was later included in the collected volume *Gender Blending* published in 1997. I cite the 1997 pagination here.

5   The American consumer movement of the 1960s also spurred the move away from medical paternalism, calling for a shift of responsibility away from omnipotent doctors to patients qua consumers.

6   For more thorough arguments about the emergence of *transgender* as a linguistic and identity category, see Califia 1997; Meyerowitz 2002; Roebuck 2013; Stryker 2008; Valentine 2007.

7   Though I met or was introduced to patients in a number of ways, my path to the clinical exam space typically began in the office lobby. After patients checked in with the receptionist, they were given information about my research project to read while they waited in the lobby. I observed clinical exams only after patients had read about the project and given verbal consent to my presence. Subsequent interviews were consented to separately.

8   Foucault (1973) has ascribed to the clinical gaze the power of creation: what is visible to the doctor is thereby made real. In Ousterhout's telling, maleness is taken to be a pure fact of human difference, preexisting the political circumstances of trans-identities and more stable than the vicissitudes of aesthetic tastes. These other things change, but maleness does not. It is there in the bones. *And you can see it.*

9   Conference presentations were important means by which surgeons attracted and met with prospective patients. Some surgeons booked almost one-third of their annual revenue through conference consultations. Following presentations, prospective patients could schedule individual consultations in surgeons' hotel rooms or be invited to private parties in surgeons' suites, where past patients shared their stories and displayed postoperative results. Conferences were not only a boon to surgeons. Prospective patients took advantage of having several far-flung surgeons

in one location and used the short consultations as a convenient way to gather information that was otherwise difficult to access.

10 There is more work to do and more questions to ask about racial and ethnic differences in the practice of FFS. During my time in the surgical clinic, patients' facial features were rarely described as having any racial or ethnic specificity. Instead they were regarded as primarily masculine or feminine—it was their face's sexually distinct characteristics that patients were there to change. Though surgeons acknowledged that facial features contain ethnic and racial connotations, there were only three occasions in the exam room during which a patient's facial features were explicitly discussed as racially or ethnically specific. The scarcity of this discussion should not be understood as a simple reflection of the overwhelming whiteness of the patient population. While it is true that the majority of patients I encountered in the clinical space identified themselves as white and were recognizably white to me, in the FFS clinic "ethnic" was not a catch-all category for nonwhiteness. Instead "ethnic" features were those that patients and surgeons both linked to a particular group and that they identified as being essentially at odds with an animating ideal of aesthetic femininity. These included some groups that are often included in the category "white," such as those with Greek and Irish ancestry. As particular features were identified and singled out as troublingly ethnic—such as one patient's Greek nose and another's Irish ears—the feminine ideal to which patients aspired grew ever more narrow. This narrowing occurred even while the logic of FFS depended on and reproduced an understanding of morphological sex difference as both binary and universal. In practice the "men look like this and women look like that" narratives of facial sex difference were both refused by the necessity of accounting for racial and ethnic difference and were reinforced through surgical plans that rendered race and ethnicity isomorphic with masculinity.

11 For a discussion and literature review of patient and surgeon expectations when using imaging software, see Agarwal et al. 2007.

3. · Cutting as Caring

1 It is an unfortunate reality that quality medical and surgical care has been hard to find. Studies consistently show that trans- people are mistreated by physicians, given inadequate care, or denied care altogether. In 2010 a national survey of over six thousand transgender and gender-nonconforming adults found that almost half (48 percent) of respondents delayed seeking medical services because they could not afford them; nearly a third (28 percent) postponed care because of feared or experienced discrimination. Of those who sought care, 19 percent reported that they'd been refused treatment because of their nonconforming gender status, and 50 percent reported the need to teach their health care provider about their medical needs (Grant et al. 2010). In the same year another survey found that when interacting with medical professionals trans- Americans experienced insensitivity to their gender of choice, practitioners' overt displays of discomfort, denial of services, substandard care, verbal abuse, and forced interventions that they did not

want (Kosenko et al. 2013). A 2010 survey found that the prevalence of health care provider mistreatment of trans- patients was twice that of gay, lesbian, or bisexual patients, and 90 percent of trans- people believed there were not enough physicians adequately trained to treat them (Lambda Legal 2010).

2 Julie K. Brown, "How Investigators Tracked Down a 'Doctor' Accused of Giving Toxic Butt Injections," *Sun Sentinel*, November 19, 2011, http://articles.sun-sentinel.com/2011-11-19/news/sfl-oneal-ron-morris-butt-injection-cement-20111119_1_injections-transgender-woman-buttocks.

3 Gary Nelson, "New Victim Reveals Fake Doc's Alleged Work," cbs *Miami*, November 28, 2011, http://miami.cbslocal.com/2011/11/28/new-victim-reveals-fake-docs-alleged-work/.

4 Laura Rena Murray, "The High Price of Looking Like a Woman," *New York Times*, August 19, 2011, http://www.nytimes.com/2011/08/21/nyregion/some-transgender-women-pay-a-high-price-to-look-more-feminine.html?pagewanted=all.

5 See Kulick (1998) for a vivid ethnographic depiction of the practice of peer-networked silicone injection in Brazil.

6 Paul Ciotti, "Why Did He Cut Off That Man's Leg? The Peculiar Practice of Dr. John Ronald Brown," *LA Weekly*, December 15, 1999.

7 Self-demand amputation has a long and complicated relationship to transsexualism (Perpich 2005; Stryker and Sullivan 2009; Sullivan 2005, 2008). In this story, however, patients are unfortunately linked by the same poor practitioner.

8 Ciotti, "Why Did He Cut Off That Man's Leg?"

9 Gold's use of the term *gender confirming facial surgery* is another example of how he is attempting to establish his ethical relationship to ffs, as well as transsexualism and gsrs more generally. gsrs is referred to by many different names, each of which carries distinct political stakes. Other than gsrs, the two most common are gender-reassignment surgery and gender-affirmation surgery. By calling his facial surgery "gender confirming facial surgery" Gold is asserting that facial bone and soft tissue reconstruction is essentially an intervention in gender and that this intervention is a confirmation of a gender that already exists and is simply being substantiated in the new face.

10 On the website *Post-Op Living*.

11 Comments on Ousterhout's website, http://www.drdouglasousterhout.com, accessed February 28, 2011.

12 I was not able to interview Shelby. Ousterhout's reports of her feelings are the only information I have regarding her assessments of her surgical results. Judging by the fact that she returned to Ousterhout for revisions after seeing Crabtree, I take his characterizations to be reasonably accurate.

4 · Recognition and Refusal

1 Meredith Jones (2009:174) has warned against thinking of patients and surgeons as working in what she calls a "simple binary relationship." To do so ignores the other kinds of players and forms of knowledge that inform this relationship and give it

shape. "Not only do these lines of analysis risk recreating the dichotomy that they describe," she writes, "they also keep the action focused on the simple dyad of doctor/patient: there is a closed, two-handed relationship here at best, and at worst the patient is also obscured, leaving only the heroic doctor standing, sweating and laboring for his own glory" (186). As powerful and often intimate as the relationships between doctors and patients were in my field site, the surgery has effects that can and do extend far beyond them.

2   While I have emphasized the conflict between visible gender transgression and being recognized as a woman in order to show how it shapes patients' relationships to the project of FFS, it is also important to remember that these positions are not homogeneous and not always mutually exclusive. Though some FFS patients wanted the surgery in order to pass and leave their trans- life and identity behind, many did not plan to "disappear" completely. They wanted to remain engaged in their trans- communities and to exercise the political power of claiming their trans- identity, but they wanted FFS to enable them to do what Maya could do, to be in control of when and how they managed this personal information. Without surgery they were out all the time, whether they wanted to be or not. It made mundane tasks like going to the grocery store difficult. It was one thing to be recognized as female and then refuse that privilege through strategic outing; it was another to not have that option at all.

3   As Toby Beauchamp (2009:363) has argued, however, "the recourse to strategic visibility remains grounded in assumptions that invisibility was ever possible. Which bodies can choose visibility, and which bodies are always already visible—perhaps even hyper-visible—to state institutions?" It is not a person's status as trans- that causes problems at airports and in police interactions; it is that they *look* trans-, that they're visibly gender-incongruent. It is also the case that people of color are more routinely stopped and questioned, flagged as being always already suspicious bodies.

4   The long-standing exclusion of trans- surgery from Medicare benefits coverage impacts the process of altering documents as well. Because surgeries are expensive and not eligible for insurance benefits, the requirement that an individual has surgery in order to change sex on legal documents has had a disproportionately adverse effect on low-income individuals. Gehi and Arkles (2007:8) write, "Medicaid exclusions of transition-related health care often not only deny low-income transgender people their only means of access to necessary treatment but also deny their only means of access to legal recognition of their identity and rights."

5   In their review of policies across the United States, van Anders and colleagues (2014:182) found, "The most common requirements [to change birth certificates is] proof of SRS [sex-reassignment surgery], followed by a surgeon's letter, and then much more distantly a letter from an MD not otherwise specified, highlighting the privileging of surgico-medical authority even over other forms of non-surgical medical authority. For [driver's licenses], the most common requirements were an MD letter, proof of SRS, a surgeon letter, and then more distantly proof of living full-time as current gender/sex, highlighting the privileging of both medical and surgico-medical authority."

6   When no particular surgery is named, "the absence of a specifier is typically under-
    stood to denote genital SRS rather than choose-your-own SRS" (van Anders et al.
    2014:182).

7   According to the National Transgender Discrimination Survey, conducted in 2011,
    "forty percent (40%) of [transgender respondents] who presented ID (when it was
    required in the ordinary course of life) that did not match their gender identity/
    expression reported being harassed and 3% reported being attacked or assaulted.
    Fifteen percent (15%) reported being asked to leave the setting in which they had
    presented incongruent identification" (Grant et al. 2010:139). Further, a trans-
    woman's surgical status impacts whether she is able to change the sex designation
    on her identification documents. According to the National Transgender Discrim-
    ination Survey, "Of MTFS [those who have transitioned from male-to-female] who
    have only had breast augmentation surgery, only 15% had changed their birth
    certificates; of those with breast surgery who tried, 32% were able to. Of transgen-
    der women who have had an orchiectomy or vaginoplasty, 55% have been able to
    change their birth certificate; of those who tried, 74% were able to do so" (139). Of
    the roughly 3,900 trans- women surveyed, 17 percent (or about 660 individuals)
    reported having had facial feminization surgery of some kind.

8   According to the 2003 *Federal Register*, "In general, an NCD is a national policy
    statement granting, limiting, or excluding Medicare coverage for a specific medical
    item or service. Often, an NCD is written in terms of a particular patient population
    that may receive (or not receive) Medicare reimbursement for a particular item or
    service. An NCD is binding on all Medicare carriers, fiscal intermediaries . . . qual-
    ity improvement organizations . . . health maintenance organizations . . . competi-
    tive medical plans . . . and health care prepayment plans" (U.S. Government 2003).

9   Following shifts in American health care management in the 1970s, "the power
    of insurers to determine coverage potentially gives them the power to dictate pro-
    fessional standards of care for all but the wealthiest patients" (Rosenbaum et al.
    1999:229). In the case of trans- surgery, a lack of robust clinical research (see Mon-
    strey et al. 2009) and the late establishment of standards of care meant little con-
    straint on American insurance providers' power to deny coverage for trans-related
    medical and surgical services.

10 The transsexualism diagnosis was replaced with gender identity disorder in the
    DSM-IV in part because clinicians wanted to separate the clinical diagnosis of trans-
    sexualism from the criteria approving people for genital sex-reassignment surgery
    (Bradley et al. 1991; Levine 1989). The new diagnostic category, gender identity
    disorder, did not compel any particular form of treatment since it was designed to
    categorize a large number of "gender dysphorias," only a fraction of which would be
    recognizable as what had been classified until 1994 as transsexualism (Pauly 1992).

11 Though diagnostic terminologies and even the continued existence of gender-
    related diagnoses have been points of contention among activists, a 2010 survey
    suggested that American trans- people were in favor of keeping *DSM* diagnosis for
    the simple reason that it is needed to access subsidized medical and surgical care
    through insurers (Vance et al. 2010).

12 New York State Register, 2014, p. 2.

13 Over time some patients notice that their lower jaw can reacquire some of the squareness they find troubling. Mira, Ousterhout's longtime assistant, noted that as faces age and soft tissues thin out, the bony structure beneath becomes more visible. This increased visibility can drive patients to request revision. Whether it was a reacquisition of bone or the thinning of her face with age, Cece was back in the office hoping to regain the tapered jaw that she had after her first operation.

14 Recent scholarship has challenged as overly reductive the portrayal of cosmetic surgery as simple and superficial. Like many trans- people, people who have plastic surgery claim that those procedures alleviate psychological suffering (Davis 2003a; Gilman 1998; Haiken 1997) and provide a means by which they can materialize the "real me" that their undesirable body obscures (Huss-Ashmore 2000; Throsby 2008).

15 Nearly all patients try to differentiate themselves from the image of the vain and preening cosmetic surgery patient. The sociologist Debra Gimlin (2010:57) calls these imagined patients "surgical others," "that is, women, whether real or imagined, whose relationship with cosmetic procedures is at best, problematic and at worst, pathological." Whereas boundary work is often done to distance "reasonable" patients from the abject figure of the "surgical junkie" (Pitts-Taylor 2007), FFS patients sought to assert a distinction between unnecessary surgeries simply meant to improve appearance and deeply needed ones that Cece described as allowing people to "engage in life."

5 · The Operating Room

1 This is not an inevitable result of facial electrolysis. Pockmarks are produced by inexperienced or unskilled technicians.

2 These procedures are a productive contrast to literature on surgery that argues that a measure of depersonalization and objectification is accomplished specifically by covering the face (Collins 1994; Goffman 1961; Hirschauer 1991; Katz 1981; Lynch 1994; Young 1997).

3 A growing body of literature elaborates this theme. See, for example, Barad 2015; Chen 2012; Hayward 2010; Hayward and Weinstein 2014; O'Brien 2013; Prosser 1998; Stryker 1994; Sullivan 2006.

4 See Halberstam (1994) on the consequences of portraying transsexualism as costuming.

5 Criticisms against the evacuation of the body were leveled by others besides trans-people of course. Indeed the most frequent criticism was the claim that Butler's theory ignores the material. The feminist scholar Vicky Kirby (1997:102) describes this position succinctly: "Critics of postmodernism warn against the effects of presuming to dissolve matter in an acid bath of rhetoric, for even if the mediated or constructed nature of reality is granted, the pressing facts of bodily existence still endure. The fear is that if the stuff of matter is problematized, or perhaps even lost, then the anchor of political contestation is also cast adrift."

6 Prosser's formulation is akin to what Oliver Sacks (1990) has called "bodily agnosia."

7 Pamela, a trans- woman with whom I shared many wonderful hours of conversation over a long weekend, was very interested in biological and physiological theories about the origins of transsexualism. "Because it *feels* physiological" was her explanation.

8 Salamon (2010) turns to psychoanalytic and phenomenological theories to consider how these models offer a way to conceive of transgender body and subject formation that is not based in their status as pathologies or as exceptions meant to prove other, ostensibly more important rules (e.g., Kessler and McKenna 1978). Salamon provides a generative and thoughtful rereading of these archives but remains concerned with figuring the body through subjecthood. In other words, for her the body is always a secondary effect—or symptom—of more fundamental psychic and epistemological realities.

REFERENCES

Adams, Vincanne, Michelle Murphy, and Adele Clark. 2009. Anticipation: Techno-science, Life, Affect, Temporality. *Subjectivity* 28(1): 246–65.

Agarwal, Anurag, Edward Gracely, and William E. Silver. 2007. Realistic Expectations: To Morph or Not to Morph? *Plastic and Reconstructive Surgery* 119(4): 1343–51.

Alexander, T. L., and H. P. Hitchcock. 1978. Cephalometric Standards for American Negro Children. *American Journal of Orthodontics* 74(3): 298–304.

Altemus, L. A. 1960. A Comparison of Cephalofacial Relationships. *Angle Orthodontist* 30(4): 223–40.

Altman, K. 2012. Facial Feminization Surgery: Current State of the Art. *International Journal of Oral and Maxillofacial Surgery* 41(8): 885–94.

American Society for Aesthetic Plastic Surgery (ASAPS). 1997. *ASAPS 1997 Statistics on Cosmetic Surgery*. New York: American Society for Aesthetic Plastic Surgery, Inc.

American Society of Plastic Surgeons (ASPS). 2014. *2014 Plastic Surgery Statistics Report*. Arlington Heights, IL: ASPS National Clearinghouse of Plastic Surgery Procedural Statistics.

Andreu, Y., and R. A. Mollineda. 2008. On the Complementarity of Face Parts for Gender Recognition. In J. Ruiz-Shulcloper and W. G. Kropatsch, eds., *Progress in Pattern Recognition, Image Analysis and Applications*, 252–60. Berlin: Springer.

Atkinson, Spencer. 1963. An Unexplored Field of Communication. *American Journal of Orthodontics* 49(8): 588–92.

Aultman, B. 2014. Cisgender. *Transgender Studies Quarterly* 1(1–2): 61–62.

Austin, John L. 1962. *How to Do Things with Words*. Cambridge, MA: Harvard University Press.

Balint, John, and Wayne Shelton. 1996. Regaining the Initiative: Forging a New Model of the Patient-Physician Relationship. *Journal of the American Medical Association* 275(11): 887–91.

Barad, Karen. 2015. Transmaterialities: Trans*/Matter/Realities and Queer Political Imaginings. *GLQ* 21(2–3): 387–422.

Bauman, Richard, and Charles L Briggs. 1990. Poetics and Performance as Critical Perspectives on Language and Social Life. *Annual Review of Anthropology* 19: 59–88.

Beauchamp, Toby. 2009. Artful Concealment and Strategic Visibility: Transgender Bodies and US State Surveillance after 9/11. *Surveillance and Society* 6(4): 356–66.

Becking, A. G., D. B. Tuinzing, J. J. Hage, and L. J. G. Gooren. 1996. Facial Corrections in Male to Female Transsexuals: A Preliminary Report on 16 Patients. *Journal of Oral and Maxillofacial Surgery* 54: 413–18.

———. 2007. Transgender Feminization of the Facial Skeleton. *Clinics in Plastic Surgery* 34(3): 557–64.

Benedict, Ruth. 1939. Sex in Primitive Society. *American Journal of Orthopsychiatry* 9: 570–73.

Benjamin, Harry. 1954. Transsexualism and Transvestism as Psycho-Somatic and Somato-Psychic Syndromes. *American Journal of Psychotherapy* 8: 219–30.

———. 1966. *The Transsexual Phenomenon.* New York: Julian Press.

Berger, Anne Emmanuelle. 2014. *The Queer Turn in Feminism: Identities, Sexualities, and the Theater of Gender.* New York: Fordham University Press.

Blakey, Michael L. 1987. Skull Doctors: Intrinsic Social and Political Bias in the History of American Physical Anthropology with a Special Reference to the Work of Ales Hrdlicka. *Critique of Anthropology* 7(2): 7–35.

Blum, Virginia L. 2003. *Flesh Wounds: The Culture of Cosmetic Surgery.* Berkeley: University of California Press.

———. 2005. Becoming the Other Woman: The Psychic Drama of Cosmetic Surgery. *Frontiers: A Journal of Women Studies* (26)2: 104–31.

Bolin, Anne. 1988. *In Search of Eve: Transsexual Rites of Passage.* South Hadley, MA: Bergin and Garvey.

Bordo, Susan. 1993. *Unbearable Weight: Feminism, Western Culture, and the Body.* Berkeley: University of California Press.

———. 1997. *Twilight Zones: The Hidden Life of Cultural Images from Plato to OJ.* Berkeley: University of California Press.

Bornstein, Kate. 1994. *Gender Outlaw: On Men, Women, and the Rest of Us.* New York: Vintage.

Boswell, Holly. 1997. The Transgender Paradigm Shift toward Free Expression. In Bonnie Bullough, Vern L. Bullough, and James Elias, eds., *Gender Blending*, 53–57. Amherst, NY: Prometheus.

Bourdieu, Pierre. 1991. *Language and Symbolic Power.* Cambridge, MA: Harvard University Press.

Bowman, C., and J. Goldberg. 2006. *Care of the Patient Undergoing Sex Reassignment Surgery.* Vancouver: Vancouver Coastal Health, Transcend Transgender Support and Education Society, and Canadian Rainbow Health Coalition.

Bradley, S., R. Blanchard, S. Coates, R. Green, S. Levine, H. Meyer-Bahlburg, I. Pauly, and K. Zucker. 1991. Interim Report of the DSM-IV Subcommittee on Gender Identity Disorders. *Archives of Sexual Behavior* 20: 333–43.

Braun, Virginia. 2009. The Women Are Doing It for Themselves: The Rhetoric of Choice and Agency around Female Genital Cosmetic Surgery. *Australian Feminist Studies* 24(60): 233–49.

Briggs, Charles L., and Daniel C. Hallin. 2007. Biocommunicability: The Neoliberal

Subject and Its Contradictions in News Coverage of Health Issues. *Social Text* 25(4): 43–66.

Brock, Dan W., and Allen E. Buchanan. 1987. The Profit Motive in Medicine. *Journal of Medicine and Philosophy* 12(1): 1–35.

Butler, Judith. 1990. *Gender Trouble*. New York: Routledge.

———. 1993. *Bodies That Matter*. New York: Routledge.

———. 1999. *Gender Trouble*. 2nd edition. New York: Routledge.

———. 2004. *Undoing Gender*. New York: Routledge.

———. 2005. *Giving an Account of Oneself*. New York: Fordham University Press.

Califia, Pat. 1997. *Sex Changes: The Politics of Transgenderism*. San Francisco: Cleis.

Cameron, Loren. 1996. *Body Alchemy*. Berkeley, CA: Cleis.

Cantú, Lionel. 2009. *The Sexuality of Migration: Border Crossings and Mexican Immigrant Men*. New York: New York University Press.

Chase, Cheryl. 1998. Hermaphrodites with Attitude: Mapping the Emergence of Intersex Political Activism. *GLQ: A Journal of Lesbian and Gay Studies* 7(4): 621–36.

Chen, Mel Y. 2012. *Animacies: Biopolitics, Racial Mattering, and Queer Affect*. Durham, NC: Duke University Press.

Cohen-Kettenis, P. T., H. A. Delemarre-van de Waal and L. J. Gooren. 2008. The Treatment of Adolescent Transsexuals: Changing Insights. *Journal of Sexual Medicine* 5(8): 1892–97.

Cohen-Kettenis, P. T., and L. J. G. Gooren. 1999. Transsexualism: A Review of Etiology, Diagnosis and Treatment. *Journal of Psychosomatic Research* 46(4): 351–33.

Cohen-Kettenis, P. T., S. E. Schagen, T. D. Steensma, A. L. de Vries, and H. A. Delemarre-van de Waal. 2011. Puberty Suppression in a Gender-Dysphoric Adolescent: A 22-Year Follow-Up. *Archives of Sexual Behavior* 40(4): 843–47.

Colebrook, Claire. 2008. On Not Becoming Man: The Materialist Politics of Unactualized Potential. In Stacy Alaimo and Susan Hekman, eds., *Material Feminisms*, 52–84. Bloomington: Indiana University Press.

Collins, H. M. 1994. Dissecting Surgery: Forms of Life Depersonalized. *Social Studies of Science* 24(2): 311–33.

Conn, Canary. 1974. *Canary: The Story of a Transsexual*. Los Angeles: Nash.

Coogan, Kelly. 2006. Fleshy Specificity: (Re)Considering Transsexual Subjects in Lesbian Communities. In Angela Pattatuci Aragón, ed., *Challenging Lesbian Norms: Intersex, Transgender, Intersectional, and Queer Perspectives*, 17–41. Binghamton, NY: Harrington Park.

Cooley, D. R., and K. Harrison, eds. 2012. *Passing/Out: Sexual Identity Veiled and Revealed*. Burlington, VT: Ashgate.

Cotton W. N., W. S. Takano, and W. M. W. Wong. 1951. The Downs Analysis Applied to Three Other Ethnic Groups. *Angle Orthodontist* 21(4): 213–20.

Cromwell, Jason. 1999. *Transmen and FTMs: Identities, Bodies, Genders, and Sexualities*. Urbana: University of Illinois Press.

Currah, Paisley, and Lisa Jean Moore. 2009. "We Won't Know Who You Are": Contesting Sex Designations in New York City Birth Certificates. *Hypatia* 24(3): 113–35.

Currah, Paisley, and Tara Mulqueen. 2011. Securitizing Gender: Identity, Biometrics, and Transgender Bodies at the Airport. *Social Research* 78(2): 557–82.

Daly, Mary. 1978. *Gyn/Ecology: The Metaethics of Radical Feminism*. Boston: Beacon.

Davidmann, Sara. 2014. Transsexual Experiences: Photography, Gender, and the Case of the Emperor's New Clothes. In Chantal Zabus and David Coad, eds., *Transgender Experience: Place, Ethnicity, and Visibility*, 108–22. New York: Routledge.

Davidson, S. P., M. S. Clifton, W. Futrell, R. Priore, and E. K. Manders. 2000. Aesthetic Considerations in Secondary Procedures for Gender Reassignment. *Aesthetic Surgery Journal* 20(6): 477–81.

Davis, Kathy. 2003a. *Dubious Equalities and Embodied Differences: Cultural Studies on Cosmetic Surgery*. Lanham, MD: Rowman and Littlefield.

———. 2003b. Surgical Passing: Or Why Michael Jackson's Nose Makes "Us" Uncomfortable. *Feminist Theory* 4(1): 73–92.

Davy, Zowie. 2011. *Recognizing Transsexuals: Personal, Political and Medicolegal Embodiment*. Burlington, VT: Ashgate.

Dechant, Dorothy. 2000. Our Best Kept Secret: The Spencer R. Atkinson Library of Applied Anatomy. *Contact Point: The Alumni Magazine of the Dugoni School of Dentistry* 80(3): 15–19.

de Lauretis, Teresa. 1991. Queer Theory: Lesbian and Gay Sexualities. An Introduction. *differences* 3(2): iii–xviii.

Dempf, Rupert, and Alexander W. Eckertet. 2010. Contouring the Forehead and Rhinoplasty in the Feminization of the Face in Male-to-Female Transsexuals. *Journal of Cranio-Maxillofacial Surgery* 38(6): 416–22.

Denny, Dallas. 1992. The Tijuana Experience. *Alicia's Girl Talk* 4(9): 18.

———. 2002. A Selective Bibliography of Transsexualism. *Journal of Gay and Lesbian Psychotherapy* 6(2): 35–66.

Derrida, Jacques. 1988. *Limited Inc*. Evanston, IL: Northwestern University Press.

Devor, Aaron H., and Nicholas Matte. 2004. ONE Inc. and Reed Erickson: The Uneasy Collaboration of Gay and Trans Activism, 1964–2003. *GLQ: A Journal of Lesbian and Gay Studies* 10(2): 179–209.

———. 2007. Building a Better World for Transpeople: Reed Erickson and the Erickson Educational Foundation. *International Journal of Transgenderism* 10(1): 47–68.

Devor, Holly. 2002. Reed Erickson (1917–1992): How One Transsexed Man Supported ONE. In Vern Bullough, ed., *Before Stonewall: Activists for Gay and Lesbian Rights in Historical Context*, 383–92. New York: Routledge.

Downing, Lisa, Iain Morland, and Nikki Sullivan. 2015. *Fuckology: Critical Essays on John Money's Diagnostic Concepts*. Chicago: University of Chicago Press.

Drummond, R. A. 1968. A Determination of Cephalometric Norms for the Negro Race. *American Journal of Orthodontics* 54(9): 670–82.

Edkins, Jenny. 2015. *Face Politics*. New York: Routledge.

Edmonds, Alexander. 2009. "Engineering the Erotic": Aesthetic Medicine and Modernization in Brazil. In Cressida Heyes and Meredith Jones, eds., *Cosmetic Surgery: A Feminist Primer*, 152–69. Burlington, VT: Ashgate.

———. 2013. The Biological Subject of Aesthetic Medicine. *Feminist Theory* 14(1): 65–82.

Enke, A. Finn. 2013. The Education of Little Cis: Cisgender and the Discipline of Opposing Bodies. In Susan Stryker and Aren Aizura, eds., *The Transgender Studies Reader 2*, 234–47. New York: Routledge.

Epstein, Steven. 2007. *Inclusion: The Politics of Difference in Medical Research*. Chicago: University of Chicago Press.

Fabian, Anne. 2010. *The Skull Collectors: Race, Science, and America's Unburied Dead*. Chicago: University of Chicago Press.

Fausto-Sterling, Anne. 2000. *Sexing the Body: Gender Politics and the Construction of Sexuality*. New York: Basic Books.

Feinberg, Leslie. 1992. *Transgender Liberation: A Movement Whose Time Has Come*. New York: World View Forum.

———. 1998. *Trans Liberation: Beyond Pink or Blue*. Boston: Beacon.

First, Michael B. 2010. Clinical Utility in the Revision of the Diagnostic and Statistical Manual of Mental Disorders (DSM). *Professional Psychology: Research and Practice* 41(6): 465.

Foucault, Michel. 1973. *The Birth of the Clinic: An Archaeology of Medical Perception*. New York: Vintage.

Frangos, Maria. 2006. Embodied Subjectivity and the Quest for Self in Televised Narratives of Body Modification. In Nancy N. Chen and Helene Moglen, eds., *Bodies in the Making: Transgressions and Transformations*, 54–62. Santa Cruz, CA: New Pacific Press.

Fraser, Suzanne. 2003. *Cosmetic Surgery: Gender and Culture*. New York: Palgrave Macmillan.

Frost, Liz. 2005. Theorizing the Young Woman in the Body. *Body and Society* 11(1): 63–85.

Gagné, Patricia, and Deanna McGaughey. 2002. Designing Women: Cultural Hegemony and the Exercise of Power among Women Who Have Undergone Elective Mammoplasty. *Gender and Society* 16(6): 814–38.

Garber, Marjorie. 1991. *Vested Interests: Cross-Dressing and Cultural Anxiety*. New York: Routledge.

Garfinkle, Harold. 1967. *Studies in Ethnomethodology*. Englewood Cliffs, NJ: Prentice-Hall.

Gehi, Pooja S., and Gabriel Arkles. 2007. Unraveling Injustice: Race and Class Impact of Medicaid Exclusions of Transition-Related Health Care for Transgender People. *Sexuality Research and Social Policy* 4(4): 7–35.

Geller, Pamela L. 2005. Skeletal Analysis and Theoretical Complications. *World Archaeology* 37(4): 597–609.

———. 2008. Conceiving Sex Fomenting a Feminist Bioarchaeology. *Journal of Social Archaeology* 8(1): 113–38.

———. 2016. *The Bioarchaeology of Socio-Sexual Lives: Queering Common Sense about Sex, Gender, and Sexuality*. New York: Springer.

Gere, Cathy. 1999. Bones That Matter: Sex Determination in Paleodemography 1948–1995. *Studies in History and Philosophy of Biological and Biomedical Sciences* 3(4): 455–71.

Ghisleni, Lara, Alexis M. Jordan, and Emily Fioccoprile. 2016. Introduction to "Binary Binds": Deconstructing Sex and Gender Dichotomies in Archaeological Practice. *Journal of Archaeological Method and Theory* 23(3): 765–87.

Giles, E. 1964. Sex Determination by Discriminant Function Analysis of the Mandible. *American Journal of Physical Anthropology* 22(2): 129–35.

Giles, E., and O. Elliot. 1963. Sex Determination by Discriminant Function Analysis of Crania. *American Journal of Physical Anthropology* 21(1): 53–68.

Gilman, Sander. 1998. *Creating Beauty to Cure the Soul: Race and Psychology in the Shaping of Aesthetic Surgery*. Durham, NC: Duke University Press.

———. 1999. *Making the Body Beautiful: A Cultural History of Aesthetic Surgery*. Princeton: Princeton University Press.

Gimlin, Debra. 2010. Imagining the Other in Cosmetic Surgery. *Body and Society* 16(4): 57–76.

Ginsberg, Elaine K. 1996. *Passing and the Fictions of Identity*. Durham, NC: Duke University Press.

Goffman, Erving. 1961. *Encounters: Two Studies in the Sociology of Interaction*. Indianapolis, IN: Bobbs-Merrill.

———. 1963. *Stigma: Notes on the Management of Spoiled Identity*. Englewood Cliffs, NJ: Prentice-Hall.

Gooren, Louis. 2006. The Biology of Human Psychosexual Differentiation. *Hormones and Behavior* 50(4): 589–601.

Gooren, Louis J. G., and Cornelis D. Doorn. 1997. What Is Medically Necessary and What Is Needed in Some Other Sense? The Case of the Transsexual Operation. In Inez De Beaufort, Medard Hilhorst, and Søren Holm, eds., *The Eye of the Beholder: Ethics and Medical Change of Appearance*, 15–25. Oslo: Scandinavian University Press.

Gould, Stephen Jay. 1981. *The Mismeasure of Man*. New York: Norton

Grant, J. M., L. A. Mottet, J. Tanis, L. Harrison, J. Herman, and M. Keisling. 2010. *National Transgender Discrimination Survey Report on Health and Health Care*. Washington, DC: National Center for Transgender Equality and National Gay and Lesbian Task Force. http://transequality.org/PDFs/NTDSReportonHealth_final.pdf. Accessed December 9, 2014.

Green, Jamison. 1999. Look! No, Don't! The Visibility Dilemma for Transsexual Men. In Kate More and Stephen Whittle, eds., *Reclaiming Genders: Transsexual Grammars at the Fin de siècle*, 117–31. New York: Cassell.

Habal, Mutaz B. 1990. Aesthetics of Feminizing the Male Face by Craniofacial Contouring of the Facial Bones. *Aesthetic and Plastic Surgery* 14: 143–50.

Hage, J. J., A. G. Becking, F. H. de Graaf, and B. D. Tuinzing. 1997a. Gender-Confirming Facial Surgery: Considerations on the Masculinity and Femininity of Faces. *Plastic and Reconstructive Surgery* 99(7): 1799–807.

Hage, J. J., M. K. Vossen, and A. G. Becking. 1997b. Rhinoplasty as Part of Gender Confirming Surgery in Male Transsexuals: Basic Considerations and Clinical Experience. *Annals of Plastic Surgery* 39: 266–71.

Haiken, Elizabeth. 1997. *Venus Envy: A History of Cosmetic Surgery*. Baltimore: Johns Hopkins University Press.

Halberstam, Judith. 1994. Skinflick: Posthuman Gender in Jonathan Demme's *The Si-lence of the Lambs. Camera Obscura*, Fall: 37–54.

Haraway, Donna. 1989. *Primate Visions: Gender, Race, and Nature in the World of Modern Science*. New York: Routledge.

———. 1997. *Modest_Witness@SecondMillenium.FemaleMan©_Meets_OncoMouse™: Feminism and Technoscience*. New York: Routledge.

Harry Benjamin International Gender Dysphoria Association. 1979. *Standards of Care: The Hormonal and Surgical Sex Reassignment of Gender Dysphoric Persons*. Version 1. Galveston, TX: Harry Benjamin International Gender Dysphoria Association.

Hausman, Bernice. 1995. *Changing Sex: Transsexualism, Technology, and the Idea of Gender*. Durham, NC: Duke University Press.

Hayward, Eva. 2010. Spider City Sex. *Women & Performance: A Journal of Feminist Theory* 20(3): 225–51.

Hayward, Eva, and Jami Weinstein. 2014. Introduction: Tranimalities in the Age of Trans* Life. *Transgender Studies Quarterly* 2(2): 195–208.

Helmreich, Stefan. 2011. Nature/Culture/Seawater. *American Anthropologist* 113(1): 132–44.

Hirschauer, Stefan. 1991. The Manufacture of Bodies in Surgery. *Social Studies of Science* 21(2): 279–319.

———. 1998. Performing Sexes and Genders in Medical Practices. In Annemarie Mol and Marc Berg, eds., *Differences in Medicine: Unraveling Practices, Techniques, and Bodies*, 13–27. Durham, NC: Duke University Press.

Hobbs, Allyson. 2014. *A Chosen Exile: A History of Racial Passing in American Life*. Cambridge, MA: Harvard University Press.

Hochschild, Arlie Russell. 1983. *The Managed Heart: Commercialization of Human Feeling*. Berkeley: University of California Press.

Hoenig, John. 1985. Etiology of Transsexualism. In Betty W. Steiner, ed., *Gender Dysphoria*, 33–73. New York: Springer.

Hoenig, J. F. 2011. Frontal Bone Remodeling for Gender Reassignment of the Male Forehead: A Gender-Reassignment Surgery. *Aesthetic Plastic Surgery* 35(6): 1043–49.

Holliday, Ruth, and Jacqueline Sanchez Taylor. 2006. Aesthetic Surgery as False Beauty. *Feminist Theory* 7(2): 179–95.

Honneth, Axel. 1995. *The Struggle for Recognition*. Cambridge, MA: MIT Press.

Hrdlička, Aleš. 1919. *Physical Anthropology: Its Scope and Aims, Its History and Present Status in the United States*. Philadelphia: Wistar Institute of Anatomy and Biology.

Huss-Ashmore, Rebecca. 2000. The Real Me: Therapeutic Narrative in Cosmetic Surgery. *Expedition* 42(3). http://penn.museum/sites/body_modification/index.html. Accessed November 15, 2010.

Irvine, Janice. 1990. *Disorders of Desire: Sex and Gender in Modern American Sexology*. Philadelphia: Temple University Press.

Isin, Engin F. 2012. *Citizens without Frontiers*. New York: Bloomsbury.

Jeffreys, Sheila. 2014. *Gender Hurts*. New York: Routledge.

Jones, Meredith. 2009. Pygmalion's Many Faces. In Cressida Heyes and Meredith Jones, eds., *Cosmetic Surgery: A Feminist Primer*, 171–90. Burlington, VT: Ashgate.

Jordanova, Ludmilla. 1989. *Sexual Visions: Images of Gender in Science and Medicine between the Eighteenth and Twentieth Centuries.* London: Harvester Wheatsheaf.

Joyce, Rosemary A. 2005. Archaeology of the Body. *Annual Review of Anthropology* 34: 139–58.

———. 2008. *Ancient Bodies, Ancient Lives: Sex, Gender, and Archaeology.* New York: Thames & Hudson.

Karkazis, Katrina. 2008. *Fixing Sex: Intersex, Medical Authority, and Lived Experience.* Durham, NC: Duke University Press.

Katz, Pearl. 1981. Ritual in the Operating Room. *Ethnology* 20(4): 335–50.

Kessler, Suzanne J., and Wendy McKenna. 1978. *Gender: An Ethnomethodological Approach.* Chicago: University of Chicago Press.

Kirby, Vicky. 1997. *Telling Flesh: The Substance of the Corporeal.* New York: Routledge.

Kosenko, Kami, Lance Rintamaki, Stephanie Raney, and Kathleen Maness. 2013. Transgender Patient Perceptions of Stigma in Health Care Contexts. *Medical Care* 51(9): 819–22.

Kotula, Dean. 2002. *The Phallus Palace: Female to Male Transsexuals.* Los Angeles: Alyson.

Kulick, Don. 1998. *Travesti.* Chicago: University of Chicago Press.

Lam, Samuel M. 2005. Aesthetic Facial Surgery for the Asian Male. *Facial Plastic Surgery* 21(4): 317–23.

Lambda Legal. 2010. *When Health Care Isn't Caring: Lambda Legal's Survey of Discrimination against LGBT People and People with HIV.* New York: Lambda Legal.

———. 2015. Changing Birth Certificate Sex Designations: State-by-State Guidelines. February 3. http://www.lambdalegal.org/publications/changing-birth-certificate-sex -designations-state-by-state-guidelines.

Laqueur, Thomas. 1990. *Making Sex.* Cambridge, MA: Harvard University Press.

Levine, Stephen B. 1989. Gender Identity Disorders of Childhood, Adolescence, and Adulthood. In H. Kaplan and B. Sadock, eds., *Comprehensive Textbook of Psychiatry,* vol. 1: 1061–69. 5th edition. Baltimore: Williams and Wilkins.

Lindqvist, Sven, 1997. *The Skull Measurer's Mistake: And Other Portraits of Men and Women Who Spoke Out against Racism.* New York: New Press.

Lorber, Judith. 1975. Good Patients and Problem Patients: Conformity and Deviance in a General Hospital. *Journal of Health and Social Behavior,* June: 213–25.

Lothstein, Leslie M. 1979. Group Therapy with Gender-Dysphoric Patients. *American Journal of Psychotherapy* 33(1): 67–81.

———. 1982. Sex Reassignment Surgery: Historical, Bioethical and Theoretical Issues. *American Journal of Psychiatry* 139(4): 417–26.

Lynch, Michael. 1994. Collins, Hirschauer and Winch: Ethnography, Exoticism, Surgery, Antisepsis and Dehorsification. *Social Studies of Science* 24(2): 354–69.

MacKenzie, Gordene Olga. 1994. *Transgender Nation.* Bowling Green, OH: Bowling Green State University Popular Press.

Markowitz, Stephanie. 2008. Change of Sex Designation on Transsexuals' Birth Certificates: Public Policy and Equal Protection. *Cardozo Journal of Law and Gender* 14: 705–30.

Martin, Biddy. 1994. Sexualities without Genders and Other Queer Utopias. *diacritics* 24(2/3): 104–21.

Martino, Mario. 1977. *Emergence: A Transsexual Autobiography*. New York: Crown.

May, William F. 1997. Money and the Medical Profession. *Kennedy Institute of Ethics Journal* 7(1): 1–13.

McBride, Cillian. 2013. *Recognition*. Cambridge: Polity.

McQueen, Paddy. 2015. *Subjectivity, Gender and the Struggle for Recognition*. New York: Palgrave Macmillan.

Mead, Margaret. (1935) 2001. *Sex and Temperament*. New York: HarperCollins.

Meadow, Tey. 2010. "A Rose Is a Rose": On Producing Legal Gender Classifications. *Gender and Society* 24(6): 814–37.

Meindl, R. S., C. O. Lovejoy, R. P. Mensforth, and T. J. Barton. 1985. Multifactorial Determination of Skeletal Age at Death: A Method and Blind Tests of Its Accuracy. *Journal of Physical Anthropology* 68(1): 1–14.

Meyer, Jon K., and Donna J. Reter. 1979. Sex Reassignment: Follow-Up. *Archives of General Psychiatry* 36(9): 1010–15.

Meyerowitz, Joanne. 2002. *How Sex Changed: A History of Transsexuality in the United States*. Cambridge, MA: Harvard University Press.

Milligan, Christine, and Andrew Power. 2010. The Changing Geography of Care. In Tim Brown, Sarah McLafferty, and Graham Moon, eds., *A Companion to Health and Medical Geography*, 567–86. New York: Wiley Blackwell.

Miravel, Julien. 2008. The Physical Examination in Cosmetic Surgery: Communication Strategies to Promote the Desirability of Surgery. *Health Communication* 23: 153–70.

Mol, Annemarie. 2002. *The Body Multiple: Ontology in Medical Practice*. Durham, NC: Duke University Press.

———. 2008. *The Logic of Care: Health and the Problem of Patient Choice*. New York: Routledge.

Mol, Annemarie, and Marc Berg. 1994. Principles and Practices of Medicine. *Culture, Medicine and Psychiatry* 18(2): 247–65.

Mol, Annemarie, and John Law. 1994. Regions, Networks and Fluids: Anaemia and Social Topology. *Social Studies of Science* 24(4): 641–71.

Monstrey, S., H. Vercruysse Jr., and G. De Cuypere. 2009. Is Gender Reassignment Surgery Evidence Based? Recommendation for the Seventh Version of the WPATH Standards of Care. *International Journal of Transgenderism* 11(3): 206–14.

Montagu, M. Ashely. 1944. Ales Hrdlicka, 1869–1943. *American Anthropologist* 46(1): 113–17.

Morgan, Kathryn Pauly. 1991. Women and the Knife: Cosmetic Surgery and the Colonization of Women's Bodies. *Hypatia* 6(2): 25–53.

Morreim, E. Haavi. 1995. *Balancing Act: The New Medical Ethics of Medicine's New Economics*. Washington, DC: Georgetown University Press.

Morrison, S. D., K. S. Vyas, S. Motakef, K. M. Gast, M. T. Chung, V. Rashidi, T. Satterwhite, W. Kuzon, and P. S. Cederna. 2016. Facial Feminization: Systematic Review of the Literature. *Plastic and Reconstructive Surgery* 137(6): 1759–70.

Nangeroni, Nancy R. 1997. SRS Tomorrow: The Physical Continuum. In Bonnie Bullough, Vern L. Bullough, and James Elias, eds., *Gender Blending*, 344–51. New York: Prometheus Books.

Newton, Esther. 1972. *Mother Camp*. Chicago: University of Chicago Press.

———. 2000. *Margaret Mead Made Me Gay: Personal Essays, Public Ideas*. Durham, NC: Duke University Press.

New York State Register. 2014. Transgender Related Care and Services. ID No. HLT-50-14-00001-P. December 17. http://docs.dos.ny.gov/info/register/2014/ dec17 /pdf/rulemaking.pdf.

Nouraei, S. A. Reza, Prem Randhawa, Peter J. Andrews, and Hesham A. Saleh. 2007. The Role of Nasal Feminization Rhinoplasty in Male-to-Female Gender Reassignment. *Archives of Facial Plastic Surgery* 9(5): 318–20.

Obedin-Maliver, Juno, Elizabeth S. Goldsmith, Leslie Stewart, William White, Eric Tran, Stephanie Brenman, Maggie Wells, David M. Fetterman, Gabriel Garcia, and Mitchell R. Lunn. 2011. Lesbian, Gay, Bisexual, and Transgender-Related Content in Undergraduate Medical Education. *Journal of the American Medical Association* 306(9): 971–77.

O'Brien, Michelle. 2013. Tracing This Body: Transsexuality, Pharmaceuticals, and Capitalism. In Susan Stryker and Aren Aizura, eds., *The Transgender Studies Reader 2*, 56–65. New York: Routledge.

Ochoa, Marcia. 2014. *Queen for a Day: Transformistas, Beauty Queens, and the Performance of Femininity in Venezuela*. Durham, NC: Duke University Press.

Ohle, John M. 2004. Constructing the Trannie: Transgender People and the Law. *Journal of Gender, Race and Justice* 8: 237.

Ousterhout, Douglas K. 1987. Feminizing of the Forehead: Contour Changing to Improve Female Aesthetics. *Plastic and Reconstructive Surgery* 79(5): 701–13.

Patton, Cindy, ed. 2010. *Rebirth of the Clinic: Places and Agents in Contemporary Health Care*. Minneapolis: University of Minnesota Press.

Pauly, Ira B. 1992. Terminology and Classification of Gender Identity Disorders. *Journal of Psychology and Human Sexuality* 5(4): 1–14.

Peltier, Bruce, and Lola Giusti. 2008. Commerce and Care: The Irreconcilable Tension between Selling and Caring. *McGeorge Law Review* 39: 785.

Perpich, Diane. 2005. Corpus Meum: Disintegrating Bodies and the Ideal of Integrity. *Hypatia* 20(3): 75–91.

Pitts, Victoria. 2006. The Body, Beauty, and Psychosocial Power. In Nancy N. Chen and Helene Moglen, eds., *Bodies in the Making: Transgressions and Transformations*, 28–46. Santa Cruz, CA: New Pacific.

Pitts-Taylor, Victoria. 2007. *Surgery Junkies: Wellness and Pathology in Cosmetic Culture*. New Brunswick, NJ: Rutgers University Press.

Plemons, Eric. 2014. Description of Sex Difference as Prescription for Sex Change: On the Origins of Facial Feminization Surgery. *Social Studies of Science* 44(5): 657–79.

———. 2015. Anatomical Authorities: On the Epistemological Exclusion of Trans- Surgical Patients. *Medical Anthropology* 34(5): 425–41.

Pollock, H. C. 1969. The Atkinson Library of Applied Anatomy. *American Journal of Orthodontics* 55(5): 510–15.

Poompruek, Panoopat, Pimpawun Boonmongkon, and Thomas E. Guadamuz. 2014. "For Me . . . It's a Miracle": Injecting Beauty among Kathoeis in a Provincial Thai City. *International Journal of Drug Policy* 25(4): 798–803.

Povinelli, Elizabeth. 2002. *The Cunning of Recognition*. Durham, NC: Duke University Press.

Prentice, R. 2012. *Bodies in Formation: An Ethnography of Anatomy and Surgery Education*. Durham, NC: Duke University Press.

Prosser, Jay. 1995. No Place Like Home: The Transgendered Narrative of Leslie Feinberg's Stone Butch Blues. *MFS Modern Fiction Studies* 41(3): 483–514.

———. 1998. *Second Skins: The Body Narratives of Transsexuality*. New York: Columbia University Press.

———. 1999. Transsexual Travelogues. In Kate More and Stephen Whittle, eds., *Reclaiming Genders: Transsexual Grammars at the Fin de siècle*, 83–114. New York: Cassell.

Rabinow, Paul. 1996. *Essays on the Anthropology of Reason*. Princeton: Princeton University Press.

Raymond, Janice. 1979. *The Transsexual Empire: The Making of the She-Male*. Boston: Beacon.

Reay, Barry. 2014. The Transsexual Phenomenon: A Counter-History. *Journal of Social History* 47(4): 1042–70.

Restack, R. M. 1979. The Sex-Change Conspiracy. *Psychology Today* 13: 20–24.

Richardson, Elijah R. 1980. Racial Differences in Dimensional Traits of the Human Face. *Angle Orthodontist* 50(4): 301–11.

Riolo, Michael, Robert E. Moyers, and James A. McNamara. 1974. *An Atlas of Craniofacial Growth: Cephalometric Standards from the University School Growth Study*. Ann Arbor: University of Michigan Center for Human Growth and Development.

Robinson, Amy. 1994. It Takes One to Know One: Passing and Communities of Common Interest. *Critical Inquiry* 20(4): 715–36.

Roebuck, Christopher W. 2013. "Workin' It": Trans* Lives in the Age of Epidemic. PhD dissertation, University of California, Berkeley.

Rose, Nicolas. 2007. *The Politics of Life Itself: Biomedicine, Power, and Subjectivity in the Twenty-First Century*. Princeton: Princeton University Press.

Rosenbaum, Sara, D. M. Frankford, B. Moore, and P. Borzi. 1999. Who Should Determine When Health Care Is Medically Necessary? *New England Journal of Medicine* 340(3): 229–32.

Rosenthal, Stephen M. 2014. Approach to the Patient: Transgender Youth. Endocrine Considerations. *Journal of Clinical Endocrinology and Metabolism* 99(12): 4379–89.

Rubin, Gayle. 1975. The Traffic in Women: Notes on the "Political Economy" of Sex. In Rayna Reiter, ed., *Toward an Anthropology of Women*, 157–210. New York: Monthly View.

———. 2002. Studying Sexual Subcultures: Excavating the Ethnography of Gay Communities in Urban North America. In Ellen Lewin and William L. Leap, eds., *Out in Theory: The Emergence of Lesbian and Gay Anthropology*, 17–68. Chicago: University of Illinois Press.

Rubin, Henry. 2003. *Self-Made Men: Identity and Embodiment among Transsexual Men*. Nashville, TN: Vanderbilt University Press.

Rudacille, Deborah. 2005. *The Riddle of Gender: Science, Activism, and Transgender Rights*. New York: Pantheon Books.

Russett, Cynthia Eagle. 1989. *Sexual Science: The Victorian Construction of Womanhood*. Cambridge, MA: Harvard University Press.

Sacks, Oliver. 1990. *The Man Who Mistook His Wife for a Hat*. New York: Harper.

Sadjadi, Sahar. 2013. The Endocrinologist's Office—Puberty Suppression: Saving Children from a Natural Disaster? *Journal of Medical Humanities* 34(2): 255–60.

Salamon, Gayle. 2010. *Assuming a Body: Transgender and Rhetorics of Materiality*. New York: Columbia University Press.

Schiebinger, Londa. 1987. Skeletons in the Closet: The First Illustrations of the Female Skeleton in Eighteenth-Century Anatomy. In Catherine Gallagher and Thomas Laqueur, eds., *The Making of the Modern Body: Sexuality and Society in the Nineteenth Century*, 42–82. Berkeley: University of California Press.

———. 1989. *The Mind Has No Sex: Women in the Origins of Modern Science*. Cambridge, MA: Harvard University Press.

———. 1993. *Nature's Body: Gender in the Making of Modern Science*. Boston: Beacon.

Schippers, Birgit. 2014. *The Political Philosophy of Judith Butler*. New York: Routledge.

Serano, Julia. 2007. *Whipping Girl: A Transsexual Woman on Sexism and the Scapegoating of Femininity*. Berkeley, CA: Seal.

Serlin, David. 2004. *Replaceable You: Engineering the Body in Postwar America*. Chicago: University of Chicago Press.

Shams, Mohammad Ghasem, and Mohammad Hosein Kalantar Motamedi. 2009. Case Report: Feminizing the Male Face. *Journal of Plastic Surgery* 9: 8–14.

Shilling, Chris. 1993. *The Body and Social Theory*. 2nd edition. London: Sage.

Shumer, Daniel E., and Norman P. Spack. 2013. Current Management of Gender Identity Disorder in Childhood and Adolescence: Guidelines, Barriers and Areas of Controversy. *Current Opinion in Endocrinology, Diabetes and Obesity* 20(1): 69–73.

Sinnott, Megan. 2004. *Toms and Dees: Transgender Identity and Female Same-Sex Relationships in Thailand*. Honolulu: University of Hawai'i Press.

Smith, Anna Marie. 1997. The Good Homosexual and the Dangerous Queer: Resisting the "New Homophobia." In Lynne Segal, ed., *New Sexual Agendas*, 214–31. London: Palgrave Macmillan.

Smith, William D. 2007. Multiculturalism, Identity, and the Articulation of Citizenship: The "Indian Question" Now. *Latin American Research Review* 42(1): 238–51.

Snow, C. C., B. P. Gatliff, and K. R. McWilliams. 1970. Reconstruction of Facial Features from the Skull: An Evaluation of Its Usefulness in Forensic Anthropology. *American Journal of Physical Anthropology* 33(2): 221–27.

Sofaer, Joanna. 2006. *The Body as Material Culture: A Theoretical Osteoarchaeology*. New York: Cambridge University Press

Somerville, Siobhan. 1994. Scientific Racism and the Emergence of the Homosexual Body. *Journal of the History of Sexuality* 5(2): 243–66.

———. 2000. *Queering the Color Line: Race and the Invention of Homosexuality in American Culture*. Durham, NC: Duke University Press.

Spade, Dean. 2003. Resisting Medicine, Re/Modeling Gender. *Berkeley Women's Law Journal* 18: 15–37.

———. 2015. *Normal Life: Administrative Violence, Critical Trans Politics, and the Limits of Law*. Durham, NC: Duke University Press.

Spiegel, Jeffrey H. 2011. Facial Determinants of Female Gender and Feminizing Forehead Cranioplasty. *Laryngoscope* 121: 250–61.

Spiegel, Jeffrey H., and Tiffiny A. Ainsworth. 2010. Quality of Life of Individuals with and without Facial Feminization Surgery or Gender Reassignment Surgery. *Quality of Life Research* 19: 1019–24.

Starr, Paul. 1982. *The Social Transformation of American Medicine*. New York: Basic Books.

Stein, Howard F. 1983. Part 1: The Money Taboo in American Medicine. *Medical Anthropology* 7(4): 1–15.

Stepan, Nancy Leys. 1986. Race and Gender: The Role of Analogy in Science. *Isis* 77(2): 261–77.

Stevenson, Lisa. 2014. *Life beside Itself*. Berkeley: University of California Press.

Stewart, T. D. 1954. Sex Determination of the Skeleton by Guess and by Measurement. *American Journal of Physical Anthropology* 12(3): 385–92.

———. 1979. *Essentials of Forensic Anthropology: Especially as Developed in the United States*. Springfield, IL: Charles T. Thomas.

St. Hoyme, Lucile E., and Mehmet Yaşar İşcan. 1989. Determinations of Sex and Race: Accuracy and Assumptions. In Mehmet Yaşar İşcan and Kenneth A. R. Kennedy, eds., *Reconstruction of Life from the Skeleton*, 53–93. New York: Alan R. Liss.

Stone, Sandy. (1991) 2006. The Empire Strikes Back: A Posttranssexual Manifesto. In Susan Stryker and Stephen Whittle, eds., *The Transgender Studies Reader*, 221–35. New York: Routledge.

Stryker, Susan. 1994. My Words to Dr. Frankenstein above the Village of Chamounix: Performing Transgender Rage. *GLQ: A Journal of Lesbian and Gay Studies* 1(3): 227–54.

———. 1999. Portrait of a Transfag Drag Hag as a Young Man: The Activist Career of Louis G. Sullivan. In Kate More and Stephen Whittle, eds., *Reclaiming Genders: Transsexual Grammars at the Fin de siècle*, 62–82. New York: Cassell.

———. 2008. *Transgender History*. Berkeley, CA: Seal.

Stryker, Susan, and Paisley Currah. 2015. Introduction. *Transgender Studies Quarterly* 2(1): 1–12.

Stryker, Susan, Paisley Currah, and Lisa Jean Moore. 2008. Introduction: Trans-, Trans, or Transgender? *WSQ* 36(3–4): 11–22.

Stryker, Susan, and Nicki Sullivan. 2009. King's Member, Queen's Body: Transsexual Surgery, Self-Demand Amputation and the Somatechnics of Sovereign Power. In Nicki Sullivan and Samantha Murray, eds., *Somatechnics: Queering the Technologisation of Bodies*, 49–64. New York: Ashgate.

Sullivan, Deborah. 2001. *Cosmetic Surgery: The Cutting Edge of Commercial Medicine in America*. New Brunswick, NJ: Rutgers University Press.

Sullivan, Nicki. 2005. Integrity, Mayhem, and the Question of Self-Demand Amputation. *Continuum: Journal of Media and Culture Studies* 19(3): 325–33.

———. 2006. Transmogrification: (Un)Becoming Others. In Susan Stryker and Stephen Whittle, eds., *The Transgender Studies Reader*, 552–64. New York: Routledge.

———. 2007. "The Price to Pay for Our Common Good": Genital Modification and the Somatechnologies of Cultural (In)Difference. *Social Semiotics* 17(3): 395–409.

———. 2008. The Role of Medicine in the (Trans) Formation of "Wrong" Bodies. *Body and Society* 14(1): 105–16.

Talley, Heather Laine. 2011. Facial Feminization Surgery: The Medical Transformation of Elective Intervention to Necessary Repair. In Jill A. Fisher, ed., *Gender and the Science of Difference: Cultural Politics of Contemporary Science and Medicine*, 189–204. New Brunswick, NJ: Rutgers University Press.

———. 2014. *Saving Face: Disfigurement and the Politics of Appearance*. New York: New York University Press.

Taylor, Charles. 1994. *Multiculturalism*. Princeton: Princeton University Press.

Thieme, F. P., and W. J. Schull. 1957. Sex Determination from the Skeleton. *Human Biology* 29(3): 242–73.

Throsby, Karen. 2008. Happy Re-Birthday: Weight Loss Surgery and the "New Me." *Body and Society* 14(1): 117–33.

Towle, Evan B., and Lynn M. Morgan. 2002. Romancing the Transgender Native: Rethinking the Use of the "Third Gender" Concept. *GLQ* 8(4): 469–97.

U.S. Department of Health and Human Services, Centers for Medicare and Medicaid Services. 2014. Chapter 1: Coverage Determinations, Part 2, Section 140.3. Transsexual Surgery. Transmittal 169, June 27. In *Medicare National Coverage Determination (NCD) Manual*. https://www.cms.gov/Regulations-and-Guidance/Guidance/Transmittals/Downloads/R169NCD.pdf.

U.S. Government. 2003. Medicare Program: Revised Process for Making National Coverage Determinations. *Federal Register* 68(107). https://www.gpo.gov/fdsys/pkg/FR-2003-09-26/pdf/03-24361.pdf.

Valentine, David. 2007. *Imagining Transgender: An Ethnography of a Category*. Durham, NC: Duke University Press.

van Anders, Siri M., N. L. Caverly, and M. M. Johns. 2014. Newborn Bio/Logics and US Legal Requirements for Changing Gender/Sex Designations on State Identity Documents. *Feminism and Psychology* 24(2): 172–92.

Vance, Stanley R., Jr., P. T. Cohen-Kettenis, J. Drescher, H. F. Meyer-Bahlburg, F. Pfäfflin, and K. J. Zucker. 2010. Opinions about the DSM Gender Identity Disorder Diagnosis: Results from an International Survey Administered to Organizations Concerned with the Welfare of Transgender People. *International Journal of Transgenderism* 12(1): 1–14.

van de Ven, B. F. M. L. 2008. Facial Feminization, Why and How? *Sexologies* 17(4): 291–98.

Van Wyhe, John. 2004. *Phrenology and the Origins of Victorian Scientific Naturalism*. Burlington, VT: Ashgate.

Vázquez, I. M., and P. M. Vila. 2006. La cirugía de reasignación sexual de hombre a mujer. *Cuadernos de Medicina Psicosomatica y Psiquiatria de Enlace* 78: 30–39.

Whitlock, Chuck. 2001. *Mediscams*. New York: St. Martin's.

Wilchins, Rikki. 1997. *Read My Lips: Sexual Subversion and the End of Gender*. Ithaca, NY: Firebrand Books.

Wittgenstein, Ludwig. (1953) 2010. *Philosophical Investigations*. New York: John Wiley and Sons.

Young, Iris Marion. 1990. *Throwing Like a Girl*. Bloomington: Indiana University Press.

Young, Katharine. 1997. *Presence in the Flesh: The Body in Medicine*. Cambridge, MA: Harvard University Press.

Zucker, K. J., P. T. Cohen-Kettenis, J. Drescher, H. F. Meyer-Bahlburg, F. Pfäfflin, and W. M. Womack. 2013. Memo Outlining Evidence for Change for Gender Identity Disorder in the DSM-5. *Archives of Sexual Behavior* 42(5): 901–14.

activism, 34, 47–49, 94, 148, 158n7
Adam's apple. *See* thyroid cartilage
aesthetics, 25, 30–32, 36, 40, 53, 61,
    64, 80–86, 130, 147, 162n8. *See also*
    beauty; facial feminization surgery
    (FFS); femininity
age. *See* youthfulness
Allure, 52
Ambulatory Surgical Clinic, 55
American Association of Orthodontists
    Foundation, 161n10
American Museum of Natural History,
    160n5
American Psychiatric Association, 45,
    102, 160n3
American Psychoanalytic Association,
    158n7
American Psychological Association,
    158n7
amputation, 73, 164n7
Arkles, Gabriel, 165n4
assimilation, 34, 99. *See also* passing;
    visibility
Atkinson, Spencer R., 31, 161n12
Atkinson Library of Applied Anatomy,
    31–32
Atlas of Craniofacial Growth, An, 29–30,
    33, 161n11
Austin, John, 9
authenticity, 15, 19, 45, 50, 63, 76,

93–95, 98, 108, 152–53. *See also*
    self-actualization

Beauchamp, Toby, 165n3
beauty, 28, 35–36, 40, 47, 57–62, 99,
    121, 131, 152. *See also* facial feminiza-
    tion surgery (FFS); femininity; race;
    youthfulness
Beck, Joel: approach to facial feminiza-
    tion surgery of, 44–45, 54–62; clinical
    strategies of, 18; early career of, 46–47;
    restitutive intimacy and, 75, 78–79, 82,
    87. *See also* beauty; facial feminization
    surgery (FFS); patient-surgeon rela-
    tionship; restitutive intimacy; surgeon
    assistants
belonging, 19, 53. *See also* recognition
Benedict, Ruth, 157n6
Benjamin, Harry, 6, 11
Berger, Anne Emmanuelle, 11–12
binary model of sex, 1–2, 33, 44–54, 64,
    96, 100, 120, 152–53, 163n10
Bloom County, 5
bodily sex, 2, 6, 9, 25, 103, 121–22,
    130–31, 154–55. *See also* genital sex-
    reassignment surgery (GSRS); sex
body, the, 2, 124–31, 148, 155–56, 168n8.
    See also facial feminization surgery
    (FFS); genital sex-reassignment sur-
    gery (GSRS); sex; social body; surgery

bone, 24, 26, 28–29, 39–42, 56–57, 103, 132, 136, 161n1. *See also* facial feminization surgery (FFS)

Boswell, Holly, 49

breast reconstruction, 3, 79, 102–5, 140

brow bossing, 40. *See also* eyebrows

brow lift, 41–42. *See also* eyebrows

Brown, John Ronald, 73–74

Butler, Judith, 9–10, 120–21, 123–24, 157n6, 158n7, 167n5

Carerra, Carmen, 99

Celebrate! (conference), 67

Center for Craniofacial Anomalies, 23

Center for Human Growth and Development, 29

cheeks, 40

chin, 4, 28–29, 33, 40–41, 52

chromosomes, 3, 16, 59, 155. *See also* bodily sex; sex

Ciotti, Paul, 73

cis-, 15, 158n9

citation, 9–10, 93

civil rights, 48. *See also* activism

clinical space, 17–19, 34, 63–66, 71, 75–87, 153, 158n11, 162n7. *See also* Beck, Joel; facial feminization surgery (FFS); Ousterhout, Douglas; restitutive intimacy

Cocoon House, 81, 137

common sense, 2–3, 10, 12, 19, 89, 100, 152

compassion, 72, 75, 78, 85, 153. *See also* patient-surgeon relationship; restitutive intimacy

conferences, 4, 30, 48, 67–69, 83, 94, 162n9

Conn, Canary, 80

consumerism, 12–13, 55, 162n5

cosmetic surgery. *See* surgery

costs, 74, 83–85, 87, 94–99, 107, 115, 130, 155. *See also* insurance

Cox, Laverne, 99

Crabtree (Doctor), 86, 164n12

Craniofacial Growth Legacy Collection, 161n10

craniofacial sex difference, 24–32, 36, 57, 130, 152, 160n8

craniofacial surgery, 5, 22, 46, 160n4

cross-dressers, 30, 67, 69, 143

Currah, Paisley, 101

Davy, Zowie, 107

Dechant, Dorothy, 31, 161n12

diagnosis, 7–8, 34, 45–46, 49–50, 102, 160n3, 166n10. *See also* transsexualism

Diagnostic and Statistical Manual of Mental Disorders, 45, 48, 160n3, 166n11

discrimination, 48, 92–93, 129–30, 144, 163n1. *See also* harassment

documentation, 16, 100–102, 108, 165n4, 166n7

Dugoni School of Dentistry, 25, 31

Edmonds, Alexander, 120

electrolysis, 23, 59, 95, 102, 116, 167n1. *See also* hair

embodiment, 114–15, 119, 123, 126, 131. *See also* gender; gender dysphoria; performativity

enactment, 6–19, 44–46, 64–66, 75, 88–91, 105–8, 121, 127–33, 152, 158n6. *See also* facial feminization surgery (FFS); femininity; recognition; womanhood

endocrine imbalance, 162n1

endocrine interventions, 3, 48, 95

Erickson Educational Foundation, 21, 160n3

essentialism, 2, 32, 35, 37, 54, 60, 100, 119, 124, 155, 158n7. *See also* gender; identity; sex

ethnography, 19, 132

eyebrows, 40–42. *See also* brow bossing; brow lift

facial feminization surgery (FFS): aims of, 48, 147–48, 152, 155; approaches to, 57–61, 64, 86; bodily sex and, 2, 9–11, 18, 30, 43, 88; cost of, 34, 84–87, 94–99, 115; criticisms of, 91–92, 97–99; definition of the female face and, 30, 36, 47, 52–54; development of, 24–29, 31–33, 161n14; disappointment with, 143–50; enactment and, 8, 18, 130, 133, 155; insurance and, 3, 48, 106–7; legal sex and, 15, 91, 99–101, 104; materiality and, 127–28; performativity and, 10–12, 15, 18, 90, 100, 154–56; procedures of, 4, 39–42, 52; race and, 26–27, 163n10; recognition and, 14–15, 44, 63, 65, 68, 90, 118, 136, 139, 154–55; restitutive intimacy and, 19, 153; self-evidence of, 5, 7, 10, 89, 142, 153; self-realization and, 13, 44, 113, 132, 141–42, 152; therapeutic legitimacy of, 50, 105, 107, 164n9; as transition, 102–6; trans- narratives and, 75–77; trans- therapeutic logics and, 7, 18, 156. *See also* Beck, Joel; common sense; enactment; female face, the; femininity; Ousterhout, Douglas; performativity; recognition; restitutive intimacy; sex; womanhood; youthfulness

facial hair, 58. *See also* electrolysis; hair

facial masculinization surgery, 109

facial sex difference. *See* craniofacial sex difference; sexual dimorphism

Federal Register, 166n8

female face, the, 23–36, 40, 43–44, 47, 53–54, 61–63, 130–31, 152, 163n10. *See also* craniofacial sex difference; facial feminization surgery (FFS); sexual dimorphism

femininity: acceptable, 17, 93; beauty and, 32, 35, 40, 53, 60, 152; definition of, 25, 29, 61, 64; ideal, 93, 152, 163n10; overall, 23, 52, 55–59, 68–69, 125, 143–49;

performative, 9–19, 88, 100, 119–32, 152–55, 158n7; race and, 25–28. *See also* beauty; facial feminization surgery (FFS); female face, the; womanhood; youthfulness

feminism, 9, 48, 158n7

forehead, 4, 28–29, 33, 40–41, 161n14

Foster, Jodie, 61

Foucault, 162n8

Fraser, Suzanne, 147

frontal sinus, 40, 52, 58

Garfinkle, Harold, 157n6

gay movement, 48

Gehi, Pooja S., 165n4

gender: aesthetics and, 32, 36; authenticity and, 13–15, 19, 45, 50, 63, 76, 93–98, 108, 152–53; binary, 96, 120, 160n6; biological theory of, 158n7; cis-, 15, 158n9; definitions of, 33, 48–49, 123–24, 131, 152, 154; hormones and, 23, 35, 45–46, 51, 95, 102–3, 115, 140; identity, 16, 47, 139; norms, 17, 92, 130; performative theory of, 9–11, 119–32, 152, 158n7; physical, 59, 103, 147, 151; recognition-based definition of, 20, 89, 107, 155; social, 8, 18, 24, 128–29; subjectivity and, 19, 122–23, 158n9; transgression, 49, 93, 96, 119–20, 122, 129, 165n2. *See also* enactment; femininity; masculinity; performativity; sex; womanhood

gender clinics, 6, 34, 48, 92, 152–53, 155, 160n2. *See also* university-based gender clinics

gender dysphoria, 22, 45–46, 51, 53, 102–3, 106, 117, 166n10

Gender Dysphoria Program (GDP), 22

gender identity disorder, 102, 166n10. *See also* gender dysphoria

genioplasty, 40

genital sex-reassignment surgery (GSRS), 1–6, 19, 23, 33–37, 73–74, 99–103, 152, 166nn7–10
Gimlin, Debra, 167n15
glabella, the, 52
Goffman, Erving, 157n6
Gold, Dr., 76, 164n9
Golden Mean, 36
gratitude, 77–80

hair, 3–4, 41, 52–53, 102, 115–16. See also electrolysis
harassment, 130, 143–46, 149, 166n7. See also violence
Hegel, Georg Wilhelm Friedrich, 15
Helmreich, Stefan, 11
HIV/AIDS, 34, 50
Honneth, Axel, 15, 93
Hoover, Herbert, 29
hormonal therapy, 23, 35, 45–46, 51, 95, 102–3, 115, 140
Hrdlička, Aleš, 160n5
Huffman, Felicity, 99
Husserl, Edmund, 126

identity, 2, 9, 19, 47, 65, 89–94, 102–8, 132, 138, 151–54, 165n2. See also authenticity; gender; gender dysphoria; politics; trans- (term)
inclusion, 98–99
individual, the, 2–3, 9, 13–19, 37, 50–51, 62–63, 90–101, 107–8, 152–56. See also identity; recognition
injections, 73–74
insurance, 3, 48, 50, 95, 101–6, 160n2, 165n4, 166n9, 166n11. See also costs
interaction, 89, 151, 155
International Journal of Sexuality and Gender Studies, 158n7
Intersex Society of North America, 34
intersubjectivity, 11–12, 20, 24, 107, 124–25
interventions, 1–8, 45–51, 64–74, 93–103, 121–23, 136, 152–55. See also facial feminization surgery (FFS); surgery; trans- medicine
invisibility, 65, 165nn2–3

jaw, 4, 41, 57, 62–63, 167n13
Johns Hopkins University, 21
Jolie, Angelina, 60
Jones, Meredith, 164n1

Kelly, Grace, 61
Kessler, Suzanne J., 157n6
Kirby, Vicky, 167n5

language, 9–10, 14, 76, 119, 124. See also narratives
Laub, Donald, 21–22, 95
lips, 4, 42. See also upper lip shortening
Lubbock, Dr., 76, 80

MacKenzie, Gordene, 48–49
malar implants, 40
"male mode," 55
maleness, 27, 40, 93, 115, 162n8. See also masculinity
male-pattern baldness, 41, 115
mandibuloplasty, 41, 52, 58
marginalization, 108. See also discrimination
marketing, 75–77, 83
Martin, Biddy, 120
Martino, Mario, 80
masculinity, 4, 9, 17, 27, 39–44, 60–63, 125, 129, 163n10, 167n13. See also femininity; gender
masseter muscle, 41
materiality, 19, 119, 121, 126–28, 130–31, 154, 167n5
maxillofacial surgery, 5, 160n4
McKenna, Wendy, 157n6
McNamara, James, 29
McQueen, Paddy, 99

Mead, Margaret, 157n6

Medicaid, 103. *See also* insurance

Medicare, 101, 103–4, 160n2, 165n4

medicine: market, 13, 45, 48, 152–53, 155; mistreatment of trans- people in, 71–72, 78, 92, 126, 163n1; paternalistic model of, 12–13, 34, 49–50, 162n5; privatization of, 12–13, 48, 102; unlicensed, 73–74, 102. *See also* surgery; trans- medicine; *specific practitioners*

mental health, 45, 160n3, 162n2

mental protuberance, 41

Merleau-Ponty, Maurice, 126

methodology, 158n11, 162n7

Meyerowitz, Joanne, 12, 80

Miami Herald, 72

Milligan, Christine, 72, 74

Mock, Janet, 99

Mol, Annemarie, 7–8, 45–46

Moore, Lisa Jean, 101

morphology, 3, 25, 29, 31, 57

Morris, Oneal Ron, 72

Morris, S. D., 62

Nangeroni, Nancy, 49–50

narratives, 12–13, 48–49, 75–77, 87, 98, 153

National Coverage Determination (NCD), 101–2

National Transgender Discrimination Survey, 166n7

Native American Graves Protection and Repatriation Act, 161n12

Newton, Esther, 158n6

New York Times, 73

normativity, 9–10, 17, 25–27, 44–45, 51–55, 61, 64–65, 93, 161n11, 161n14. *See also* craniofacial sex difference; female face, the

nose, 4, 28–29, 33, 52, 58. *See also* rhinoplasty

orthodontics, 29, 161n10

Ousterhout, Douglas: approach to FFS of, 5–6, 57, 60, 62, 132–34; beauty and, 35–36; books by, 142; conferences and, 4, 30; definition of the female face of, 30, 44, 52–55, 162n8; early career of, 21–29, 31–33, 160n8, 161n14; recognition and, 14, 65; restitutive care and, 18, 75, 77–81, 87; "wrong body" and, 50–51. *See also* Cocoon House

Ousterhout, Oliver, 36

Paltrow, Gwyneth, 60

passing, 14–15, 19, 65, 90–92, 96, 99–100, 107, 143, 152–53, 158n9, 165n2

paternalism, 34, 49–50, 92, 152, 162n5. *See also* trans- medicine

pathology, 34, 48–50, 92, 102; "wrong body" model of, 18

patient-centered treatment models, 48, 162n2

patient-surgeon relationship, 19, 70, 75, 77–80, 84, 95, 164n1. *See also* restitutive intimacy

performativity, 9–19, 88, 100, 119–32, 152–55, 158n7

Pfeiffer, Michelle, 61

physical anthropology, 24–28, 32

policy, 90, 102–3, 165n5

politics, 14, 19, 34, 66, 91–99, 108, 142, 158n9, 162n8. *See also* activism; identity; queer politics; trans- (term)

Pollock, H. C., 161n12

Povinelli, Elizabeth, 99

Power, Andrew, 72, 74

Prince, Virginia, 48–49

privatization, 12–13, 48

Prosser, Jay, 76, 108, 123–24

psychoanalytics, 162n1, 168n8

psychopathology, 48

psychotherapy, 45–46, 95

puberty, 54, 116–17

queer politics, 33, 50
queer theory, 34, 131, 160n6

race, 25–29, 32, 34, 96, 98, 152, 161n11,
    163n10
"real" body, 124–26
recognition: facial feminization surgery
    and, 15, 44, 154; legal, 99–101; as male,
    27; model of sex based on, 3, 10–12,
    90; political, 19, 91–94, 98; postoper-
    ative, 5, 63, 136, 141; sex and, 2, 24, 37;
    social, 18, 89, 107, 118, 124, 130, 152,
    156; as trans-, 143, 147, 165n3; trans-
    therapeutics and, 20; womanhood and,
    36, 54, 68, 90, 108, 129–30, 139, 149,
    151, 155. See also refusal
reconstructive surgeries. See facial femi-
    nization surgery (FFS); genital sex-
    reassignment surgery (GSRS); surgery;
    transition
redistributive justice, 93, 107–8
refusal, 15, 65, 88–108, 143–46, 149
restitutive intimacy, 19, 71–88, 152
rhinoplasty, 40, 42, 52, 86, 116. See also
    nose

Salamon, Gayle, 124–26, 168n8
San Francisco, 18, 23, 25, 33–34, 36, 46,
    51, 137
scalp, 4, 41
self-actualization, 13, 17, 51, 63, 72, 105,
    108, 151–53
self-determination, 34–35, 49–50, 92
self-evidence, 5, 7, 10, 89, 142, 153
self-optimization, 44–45, 47, 50
Serano, Julia, 14
sex: appeal, 44, 57, 61, 64; binary model
    of, 1–2, 33, 44–54, 64, 96, 100, 120,
    152–53, 160n6, 163n10; biological nar-
    rative of, 157n6, 158n7, 162n8; bodily,
    2, 6, 8–9, 25, 103, 121–22, 130–31,
    154–55; chromosomal definition of,
    3, 16; facial, 8, 26–28, 32, 37, 151;

genital definition of, 1–6, 24, 33, 47,
    99, 101, 107, 119, 132, 154; hormones
    and, 23, 35, 45–46, 51, 95, 102–3, 115,
    140; legal, 15, 19, 23, 90, 100–101,
    104, 165n4; performativity and, 120,
    124, 130, 152; recognition-based model
    of, 3, 10–12, 18, 20, 24, 37, 130, 155;
    surgery and, 33, 147. See also gender;
    sexual dimorphism
sex-differentiating characteristics, 26,
    28
sexual dimorphism, 29–36, 44, 47, 54, 64,
    121, 130, 154, 157n6, 160n8, 162n8
sexuality, 9, 158n7
sinus, 57
skin care, 59
skulls. See craniofacial sex difference
social body, 2, 124–28, 148, 155–56
social gender, 6, 11, 15–18, 23–25, 90,
    105, 125, 130, 148–56
social justice, 96
social life, 9, 14, 23, 126
soft tissue, 39–41
Somerville, Siobhan, 27
Standards of Care, 107, 160n3
Stanford University, 21. See also Gender
    Dysphoria Program (GDP)
Stone, Sandy, 92, 96, 98
Stryker, Susan, 22
subjectivity, 122–23, 158n9
surgeon assistants, 80–85
surgery: bodily sex and, 2; cosmetic, 2,
    5, 24, 30, 46, 48, 103–5, 152, 158n8,
    167nn14–15; elective, 50, 102, 104–5;
    expense of, 12, 14, 34, 74, 83–85, 87,
    94–99; genital reconstructive, 1, 35,
    62; goals of, 13, 17–18, 35, 45–46; in-
    surance and, 48, 50, 103; intervention
    and, 2, 67, 71; legal sex and, 15, 19, 23,
    90, 100–101, 104, 165n4; recognition
    and, 14, 68; restitutive intimacy and,
    71–88, 163n1; therapeutic legitimacy
    of, 1, 19, 50, 105, 107, 167n14; transfor-
    mation and, 66, 147, 155. See also facial

feminization surgery (FFS); genital sex-reassignment surgery (GSRS); transition; *specific surgeons*

Tambor, Jeffrey, 99
Taylor, Charles, 93
Tessier, Paul, 23
testosterone, 6, 41, 54. *See also* hormonal therapy
thyroid cartilage, 4, 42, 52, 109–11, 116
tracheal shave, 42. *See also* thyroid cartilage
trans- (term), 7, 16–17, 119, 157n1
TransAmerica, 99
transgender, 16, 35, 49–50, 122, 157n1
transgender public health program, 34
transgression, 93, 96, 119–20, 122, 129, 165n2
transition, 3, 14, 18, 23, 35, 44–46, 51, 95, 102–4, 115–17, 140. *See also* facial feminization surgery (FFS); genital sex-reassignment surgery (GSRS); interventions; surgery; trans- medicine
trans- medicine: access to, 95, 130; evolution of, 6, 19, 22, 34, 47, 66, 92, 151, 153, 166n9; goals of, 3, 12, 45–46, 101, 152; hormone therapy and, 23, 35, 44–45, 51, 95, 102–4, 115, 140; insurance and, 101–7, 166nn8–9, 166n11; paternalistic model of, 12–13, 49–50; patient-centered model of, 45, 63, 162n2; restitutive intimacy of, 71–88; self-determination and, 34–35, 49–50, 92; therapeutic legitimacy of, 1, 50, 105, 107, 167n14; therapeutic logics of, 4, 6–8, 19, 44–45; "wrong body" narrative and, 13, 18, 48, 50–51, 60, 63, 123, 152. *See also* clinical space; interventions; medicine; surgery; transition; trans- therapeutics
Transparent, 99
trans- people, 12–15, 45–48, 74, 91, 98, 123–30. *See also* activism; bodily sex; discrimination; gender; identity; transwomen; violence; visibility
transphobia, 94. *See also* discrimination
transsexualism, 1–2, 6–24, 33–37, 44–50, 95, 101–3, 119–22, 155, 160n3, 166n10, 168n7. *See also* politics; social body; trans- (term); transition; trans- medicine; trans- women; visibility
Transsexual Menace, 34
trans- therapeutics: genital-centric, 101–4, 132, 152; logics of, 3–8, 11–12, 18, 44, 91, 101–5, 133, 155–56; models of, 18, 45, 50–51, 107; recognition and, 10–11, 20; restitutive intimacy and, 71–72, 87
transvestitism, 6, 11
trans- women: conferences for, 4, 30, 48, 67–69, 83, 94, 162n9; narratives of, 12–13, 48–49, 75–77, 87, 98, 153; performativity and, 9–19, 88, 100, 119–32, 152–55, 158n7; recognition and, 9–10, 89, 93, 147; restitutive intimacy and, 19, 71–88, 152; visibility of, 92–99, 108. *See also* facial feminization surgery (FFS); femininity; gender; interventions; politics; recognition; surgery; transition; trans- medicine; visibility; womanhood

university-based gender clinics, 12, 21–22, 48, 160n2. *See also* gender clinics
University of California, Berkeley, 34
University of California, San Francisco, 23, 34. *See also* Center for Craniofacial Anomalies
University of Michigan, 21, 25, 28–29, 160n2
University of the Pacific, San Francisco, 25, 31
University School Growth Study (USGS), 28–30, 33, 35, 54, 161nn10–11
upper lip shortening, 42, 52–53, 57. *See also* lips

U.S. Department of Health and Human Services (DHHS), 101–2
U.S. Supreme Court, 50

van Anders, Siri M., 100, 165n5
van de Ven, Bart, 147
violence, 98, 126, 129–30. *See also* harassment
visibility, 92–99, 108
voice, 3, 103

weight, 52
womanhood: affecting, 19, 148; enactment and, 7, 14, 18, 44, 51, 66, 88, 105, 129, 134; facial feminization surgery and, 6, 11, 48, 89, 106; performative, 9–19, 88, 100, 119–32, 152–55, 158n7; recognition of, 2, 36, 90, 99, 107–8, 129–30, 139, 149, 155; refusal of, 15, 65, 88–108, 143–46, 149. *See also* femininity; gender; recognition; sex; trans- women
World Professional Association for Transgender Health, 48, 107, 162n2
World War II, 8, 26
"wrong body," 13, 18, 44, 48, 50–51, 60, 63, 123, 152

Young, Iris Marion, 93
youthfulness, 40–41, 57–59, 61, 115, 149–50

Zellweger, Renée, 61